CLIFF SHEATS
LEAN BODIES
TOTAL FITNESS

CLIFF SHEATS
LEAN BODIES
TOTAL FITNESS

Get Leaner Faster with

Fat Burning Workouts and Increased Calories

BY CLIFF SHEATS, M.S., WITH
MAGGIE GREENWOOD-ROBINSON

THE SUMMIT PUBLISHING GROUP
ARLINGTON, TEXAS

THE SUMMIT PUBLISHING GROUP

One Arlington Centre, 1112 East Copeland Road, Fifth Floor, Arlington, Texas, 76011

Copyright ©1995 by Cliff Sheats and Maggie Greenwood-Robinson.

All rights reserved. No part of this book may be reproduced or transmitted in any form or by any means, electronic or mechanical, including photocopying, recording or by any information storage and retrieval system without the written permission of the publisher, except where permitted by law. Any mention of retail products does not constitute an endorsement by the publisher.

99 98 97 96 95 5 4 3 2 1

LIBRARY OF CONGRESS CATALOGING IN PUBLICATION DATA

Sheats, Cliff.

[Lean bodies total fitness workout]

Cliff Sheats lean bodies total fitness : get leaner faster with fat burning workouts and increased calories / by Cliff Sheats, with Maggie Greenwood-Robinson.

p. cm.

Includes bibliographical references and index.

ISBN 1-56530-188-9 (Hardcover : alk. paper)

1. Reducing exercises. 2. Reducing diets. 3. Weight loss.

I. Greenwood-Robinson, Maggie. II. Title.

RA781.6.S54 1995

613.7—dc20   95-42290

                                                                CIP

Cover Design by David Sims and Jim Strickland
Book Design by David Sims
Cover photograph by Truitt Rogers
Food Styling by Patricia Fly

To Kathy, Jonathan, and Allison

In Loving Memory of Nancy G. Sheats

THE SUGGESTIONS FOR SPECIFIC FOODS, nutritional supplements, and exercise in this book are not intended as a substitute for consultation with your physician. After you have met your desired body composition goals, it is recommended that you consult with a qualified health professional to establish food intake to maintain your energy needs. Long-term usage of nutritional supplementation is not recommended unless done so under the guidance of a physician, clinical nutritionist, or registered dietitian.

Individual needs vary, and no diet, nutrition program, or exercise plan will meet everyone's daily requirements. Before starting the Lean Bodies Workout or eating program, always see your physician. The use of specific products in this book does not constitute an endorsement by the authors or the publisher.

CONTEN

T S

Acknowledgments

THE LEAN BODIES WORKOUT is a special book to me. Many years ago, I struggled with a lack of physical strength. This worried me greatly, since my wife and I wanted to someday become parents. I truly wanted to be a father, but I was too tired and weak. Something had to change. Being a man of faith, I prayed to God, asking Him for guidance in what I should do to become stronger and healthier — in order to be a good dad and to raise my children to be physically and spiritually strong. He was faithful as always, and a sequence of events transpired. God put certain people in my life to help me with my nutrition education and restoration to physical health. My transformation continued, as I began to see what direction my life would take in terms of education and later as I developed the Lean Bodies program to help others become more healthy.

Today, I am the father of two precious children, Jonathan, 5, and Allison, 2, and the husband of one of the greatest wives and mothers on earth, Kathy. God certainly answered my prayers.

First, I would like to thank my wife and children. They have been a great blessing to me. Thanks for allowing me to share in the love that God has given us for each other as a family. Kathy, you are truly a wonderful example of the "virtuous woman" in the Bible. Everyday, your gentle loving spirit is enjoyed by myself and our children. Jonathan and Allison, you guys are special gifts from God. I'm just glad He has entrusted you to me and your mom.

Heartfelt thanks go out to the Cokers, for sharing their special love with me and my family. We love you, guys! Thank you, Kathy Coker, for being my big sister. Your nurturing love has meant so much to me — you have always been there. God has given us a special love for each other. Cary, thanks for standing beside me as a brother in Christ.

Next, I thank my Mom and Dad, for their support and love throughout the years. I love you!

I also thank my brother Bob. God has truly given you great talents. I'm glad you're happily using them.

My deep thanks go to The Summit Group and the entire staff there for the foresight to publish a sequel to *Cliff Sheats Lean Bodies.*

Then of course there is Maggie Greenwood-Robinson, my friend and co-author. I am deeply indebted to Maggie for her invaluable expertise and writing skills with which God has blessed her. She is truly a great researcher and writer who made my job easy because of her "sense of excellence" to our project. Maggie has a gift to be able to take complicated subject matter and digest it into easy-to-understand material. Also, her endurance in looking up research and discernment of validity is unparalleled.

My very special thanks go to Dr. Luke Bucci, Ph.D., for his discerning eye and review of the manuscript.

As well, I am indebted to my friend and colleague John Parrillo, who brought the concept of building the metabolism to the forefront of nutritional science. His 20 years of working with athletes and bodybuilders has contributed greatly to my knowledge of sports nutrition.

Much appreciation goes to my staff: Wes Cade, for his expertise and knowledge as a professional trainer, as well as his meticulous eye for details; and Dwayne Wilson, for his assistance and input from his athletic background and experience as a professional trainer. Thanks for being my friends.

My thanks and appreciation also go to Roland Jehl, my brother in Christ, who has also stood by me. Roland has been very kind to let me be a part of his radio show on KLIF in Dallas. As anyone who has ever met Roland knows, he is of impeccable character and tells people the truth about nutrition and training. He is a warehouse of wisdom. His walk with the Lord has been an inspiration to me and to others.

Finally, I thank all my other friends, for sticking by me through my ups and downs. My love to all of you.

Please keep in mind that this workout book is good only for the time you are on this earth. I would like to encourage you to read God's inspired word, The Bible, especially if you want to know what happens after this life, whether you are bound for heaven, and, most importantly, how to be sure. I suggest the book of John, Acts 16:31, and I Corinthians 15:3-4 as starting points for anyone who seeks the spiritual surety of everlasting life.

How to Use this Book

The Lean Bodies Workout is a new, revolutionary exercise program designed specifically to help you burn body fat fast and build metabolically active muscle at the same time. If you follow the principles covered in this book, you'll be amazed by the differences in your appearance, energy levels, and overall health. You'll experience a fitness you can feel and fitness you can see.

Intellectually, most people know that exercise takes off fat pounds. But in reality, they just don't know how to exercise properly to achieve this goal. Most go about exercise in a haphazard manner, and the results are both mediocre and disheartening. The Lean Bodies Workout teaches you scientifically proven methods of fat-burning that will produce rapid results.

I have organized this book around five major parts: getting leaner and healthier, faster; moving from fat to fit in just eight weeks; fueling yourself for fat-burning and energy production; supplementing for super-charged results; and making the Lean Bodies Workout a lifestyle for a lifetime.

Under each part are chapters that cover the specifics about fat-burning exercise. Part I, for example, describes the benefits of different types of exercise and how to tap into their fat-searing power. Part II includes 10 exercise techniques that force your body to start combusting fat, along with special exercises and routines. Parts III and IV cover the all-important issue of nutrition — and how you can increase calories for maximum body fat loss and greater energy. Part V teaches you some new exercise motivation techniques.

I have also included several Appendices. Appendix A, for example, is for people who are interested primarily in gaining lean muscle, rather than losing body fat. In Appendix B, I answer questions that are on practically every exerciser's mind. For easy reference, there's an extensive glossary of terms used in this book. Finally, other appendices describe recommended products and reading material that will help you succeed on the Lean Bodies Workout.

While it's best to read this book sequentially — that is, from cover to cover — you can also skip around to easily locate the information you need. My hope is that you'll keep this book handy, as a guide and motivator. It has been my goal to make the information easy to understand, easy to find, and easy to refer to. Also, you'll want to use this book in conjunction with my two previous books, *Cliff Sheats Lean Bodies: The Revolutionary New Approach To Losing Body Fat By Increasing Calories* and *The Lean Bodies Cookbook,* both in paperback.

The information in the Lean Bodies Workout is based on the most up-to-date research from exercise science, plus numerous, real-life case studies of people who have transformed their bodies and their health by following the Lean Bodies programs. Their stories are truly incredible, and I know you'll get charged up when you read them.

My hope is that you'll join the legions of people who have made successful lifestyle changes as a result of the "Lean Bodies revolution." You have nothing to lose (except your unwanted body fat), and everything to gain in terms of a fit, active, and healthy life.

Cliff Sheats, M.S.

Part I

Get Leaner, Healthier —Faster

1

CHAPTER ONE

The Five Exercise Secrets Behind Fat Loss

INTRODUCING The Lean Bodies Workout, America —
it's time to get moving! About 27 percent of us are considered sedentary — in other words, couch potatoes —
33 percent of us are on-again off-again exercisers and 71
percent are overweight. In short, very few people get
enough exercise to burn health-ruining fat or improve
vital heart and lung fitness. It's no wonder that heart disease, obesity, and other chronic diseases are on a deadly
climb in our society.

But enough about society. What about you? Have
you tried umpteen exercise programs but without much success?
Or are you currently inactive but want to give exercise a try?
Maybe you're among the minority of Americans who do exercise
regularly, but you want to push yourself harder and farther.

Whatever your current exercise status, welcome to the Lean
Bodies Workout. I know you are asking yourself: What exactly is
the Lean Bodies Workout? In a nutshell, the workout is a revolutionary exercise system that forces your body into a fat-burning,
health-building mode — and does this fast (no waiting around
months for results). It's the first exercise program that shows
America how to work out more effectively for minimum body fat,
maximum muscle tone, and maximum health. The Lean Bodies
Workout will revolutionize the way America exercises, just like
the Lean Bodies eating program revolutionized the way we eat.

In fact, the Lean Bodies Workout is designed to go hand-in-hand with the Lean Bodies eating program, explained in my best-selling book, *Cliff Sheats Lean Bodies: The Revolutionary Approach To Losing Body Fat By Increasing Calories.* You see, one of the biggest mistakes exercisers make is not eating enough. That's right! When calories are in short supply — as they are on most restrictive diets — your metabolism downshifts so much that you can't possibly burn fat or develop lean, toned tissue. All the exercise in the world won't give you the body you want as long as your metabolism is in the basement. More on that later.

How The Lean Bodies Workout Was Created

Lean Bodies itself started in the late 1980s when I was working with a cardiologist and seeing people who had various health problems. The common denominator in most of these cases was poor nutrition. It became apparent that these people either weren't eating enough or they were filling up on the wrong foods. So I began teaching people how to increase their calories to lose body fat. Increasing calories outmaneuvers metabolic slowdown — and thus makes the body more efficient at burning body fat.

What also revs up the metabolism to burn fat is exercise, as long as you know how to maximize its fat-burning power. Exercise can have such a profound effect that my staff and I began encouraging Lean Bodies participants to "get moving." We found, however, that many people didn't know how to begin an exercise program, others were sweating and sacrificing without getting results, and some were stop/start exercisers with low motivation. Virtually no one knew how to exercise correctly to achieve the one thing we all want from exercise: Burn pure fat!

A dramatic about-face was in order. We needed a structured, motivating exercise program that would do three things: (1) Force the body into a fat-burning mode immediately so that people could see visible results fast; (2) Provide an easy-to-follow, no-fail system of exercising; (3) Work hand-in-hand with the Lean Bodies eating program to help people pursue and maintain a healthful, high-energy lifestyle. Unlike a lot of exercise programs, it integrates the biochemistry of nutrition with exercise physiology. This is a critical union, since the exercising body has to be stoked with the right fuels to incinerate fat. Nutrition and exercise physiology simply can't be separated.

Benefits Of The Lean Bodies Workout

Many people start exercising with high hopes that they'll lose body fat. Yet, they're disappointed when the results fail to materialize as expected. They may quit exercise altogether and return to a sedentary lifestyle with poor eating habits. This reaction is understandable, since few exercise programs are geared for rapid fat loss. The entire focus and design of the Lean Bodies Workout is to make your body adapt to exercise in such a way that it will effectively and rapidly process fat for energy. The fact that body fat begins to melt off within days is self-motivating. After all, who would want to quit exercising with those kinds of results? With this in mind, here's what you can expect from the Lean Bodies Workout:

• A leaner, fitter physique. You'll see visible results as rapidly as the first week of the workout.

• A racehorse metabolism. Your body becomes a fat-burning, muscle-developing machine.

• Through-the-roof energy levels. You'll re-discover just how much energy your body can really produce. Physical energy crises will become a thing of the past.

• Reduced risk factors for cardiovascular disease. Cholesterol can drop to healthy ranges, and your heart gets more efficient at doing its job.

• Postponement of the effects of aging, as you rebuild vital body tissue and aerobic power.

• An athlete-like drive to push yourself physically — and succeed at doing so.

Sound too good to be true? Hold on. Let me introduce you to some people on the Lean Bodies Workout.

Real-Life Successes

• "I was tired of carrying around 390 pounds and feeling tired all the time!" says Ron M.

So he set out to shed his excess fat baggage by changing both his diet and his sedentary lifestyle. Ron began Lean Bodies, and before long felt energetic enough to start a walking program, gradually building up to five 30-minute walks a week. The upshot of Ron's effort is that he's lost 100 pounds (including eight inches off his waist)!

• David L. had always exercised regularly, yet his body fat percentage was stuck at 17 percent, somewhat on the high side for a man. Plus, he weighed 14 pounds too many. One problem was his history of yo-yo dieting. David had been on and off calorie-restrictive diets so much that his body was literally hoarding fat.

David started Lean Bodies and before long increased his calories significantly. He learned what foods to eat to lose body fat and to stay energetic. "As a result, my energy level went up because I had plenty of 'fuel'," he says.

With his energy sky-high, David went on the Lean Bodies Workout, using the principles you will learn about shortly. As a result, he whittled his body fat down to a lean 10 percent, which he's been able to maintain.

• A reduction of two pants sizes, an increase in muscle tone, and seemingly boundless energy for sports and exercise have been the rewards of the Lean Bodies Workout for Jerry C. He was a participant in a study I'm conducting with the employees at a large corporation. "My personal physician had recommended the Lean Bodies program to me," Jerry says. "When my company offered the program to its night shift workers, I was able to participate."

Jerry needed to lose weight, plus lower his blood pressure, which was hovering at unsafe levels. A history of heart disease in his family was a motivating factor in his determination to succeed on the program.

And he did. Jerry lost body fat, reduced his blood pressure, and gained more energy. "The combination of diet and exercise has improved my stamina in playing softball and golf — especially golf. I'm no longer tired or winded after playing 18 holes. This is one program I will stay with from this day forward," he says.

• Sue S. had tried many diets, but to no avail. Then she heard about the Lean Bodies program on a radio show. She bought the first Lean Bodies book, read it, and liked the approach. Needing a support group to help her get started, Sue signed up for the Lean Bodies classes.*

*If you would like to come to a six-week course that teaches you all about Lean Bodies, call today! 1-800-697-LEAN, 1-214-380-LEAN

"I liked the concept, and it was sensible. Plus, it was something I thought my family would be able to do with me. As it turned out, the program was really helpful for all of us," Sue says.

Sue gradually increased her calories to 2,000 a day, divided into six daily meals. Her body fat began to peel off, and, at the same time, she increased her lean mass. Even her cholesterol, which was too high, moved into a healthier range.

"I'm also prone to osteoporosis and feel like the Lean Bodies Workout will be helpful in preventing that," she adds. "I'm sold on the entire program."

• Anne A. believes she has pushed herself farther than she ever thought she could, thanks to the Lean Bodies Workout. "I can deadlift [a rigorous barbell exercise] 65 pounds and do walking lunges around the track holding two 20-pound dumbbells. My legs are strong. I have a lot more confidence and mental and physical stamina.

"I like having the look of an athlete. I like the muscle definition I have and wish women wouldn't be so skeptical of weight training."

Nutritionally, Anne increased her calories and learned how to "clean up" her diet to eat foods that would convert easily into energy and muscle tissue, but not into body fat. Anne dropped several dress sizes by following the Lean Bodies Workout and eating program.

Of course, these are just a few of the many success stories I've seen at Lean Bodies. Now let's get into the five "secrets" of the Lean Bodies Workout — and why it produces such body-changing results.

SECRET #1:
Pump up your intensity.

For too many years now, exercisers and wannabe exercisers have been a little misled by reports that any type of exercise, even mild forms like gardening, golfing, and strolling in the park, is all you need to be in optimal shape. Not true! While it's fair to say that some activity is better than none, you're simply not going to develop fat-burning muscle or peak cardiovascular fitness with low-level exercise. I love to play golf, but I don't rely on it to achieve peak fitness!

You've got to perform higher-intensity exercise to get results. "Intensity" has several different meanings depending on the type of exercise you do, but it basically describes how hard you work out.

Now, before I go any further, I realize the thought of vigorous exercise is enough to make a lot of people head straight back to the couch. All I'm saying is that higher-intensity exercise produces the fat-burning, health-building results you want from exercise. This fact has been proved repeatedly by the latest research in exercise science. Studies show that people who work out harder are leaner and more toned — plus, they achieve conditioning faster. Intense exercise actually turns certain muscle fibers into fat-burning factories. Even more important, vigorous exercisers have fewer health problems, and live better, more actively.

To look at it another way: The value of low-intensity exercise can be likened to earning 10 percent on $20,000, whereas higher-intensity exercise is more like earning 3 percent on $1 million. There's just that much difference in health and fitness gains!

Does all this mean the Lean Bodies Workout is time-consuming? Not at all. Intensity doesn't necessarily correlate with time. It's the effort you give for the time you put in, whether it's 20 minutes or 45 minutes. The Lean Bodies Workout is time-efficient. In fact, some portions of the workout are performed only twice a week. You can definitely develop greater levels of fitness in a shorter period of time.

So important is intensity that I've devoted an entire chapter to it. If you're sedentary now, sporadically active, or highly active, I'll show you how to gradually increase your intensity — just like you learned to gradually increase your calories in the first Lean Bodies book — and knock fat off for good, plus be healthier for it. You will be amazed at what your body can accomplish physically.

SECRET #2:
Combine aerobic exercise and weight training.

Go into most gyms or health clubs today, and you will generally see two distinct groups of people: the aerobic exercisers and the weight trainers. To use a familiar phrase, never the twain shall meet. Not so with the Lean Bodies Workout. If you're doing one and not the other, you are only halfway home. You absolutely must do both if you want to burn fat and get in peak condition. Anyone who uses a combination of aerobic exercise and weight training burns more fat, plus builds and preserves precious muscle mass better than those who just stick to one form of exercise.

You'll learn more about the value of combination exercise throughout this book, but here's more about why this dual approach works so well:

• Double your fat-burning power. Aerobic exercise burns fat by increasing fat-burning enzymes in your body and by building your aerobic power, another factor in fat-burning. Weight training also burns fat, but in a different way — by creating metabolically active muscle tissue. Muscle tissue is fat-burning tissue.

So with combination exercise, you are burning fat not one way but two ways!

• Combination exercise changes your shape for the better. When you exercise aerobically and use weights, some remarkable things happen. You lose unwanted fat pounds, trim off inches, and reshape your body. Nothing else works as well. Typically, dieting without exercise makes you lose mostly muscle, and you still look flabby as a result. Aerobic-only exercise succeeds in burning fat, with some gains in body-firming muscle. But add weight training to aerobics, and you lose more body fat and gain more lean, fat-burning muscle. Plus, you can redistribute your weight for a more balanced physique. Your entire body changes for the better, and these changes can happen at any age, too.

• Strength and endurance improve dramatically with combination training. In one study, researchers looked into the effect of combining weight training and aerobics on aerobic capacity and strength levels. Sedentary men were divided into one of three groups: a weight training-only group, an aerobics-only group, and a combined group, which did weight training and aerobics in the same exercise session. Both the weight-trained and the combination groups increased their strength as well as their lean muscle. But none of the aerobics group improved in those two areas. Aerobic capacity improved in the aerobics and the combination group.[1] The bottom line here is that you can get the best of both worlds — strength and endurance — by performing a combination workout.

This evidence only scratches the surface of the value of combination exercise. It's simply too powerful to ignore. You must do both. Aerobic exercise and weight training each have a unique set of benefits. By doing both, you multiply the effect of exercise on your health, fitness, and overall quality of life.

Again, this doesn't mean you have to spend even more time exercising. On the Lean Bodies Workout, you learn techniques that will minimize the time you spend exercising while maximizing your fat-burning, health-building potential.

SECRET #3:
Use proven fat-burning exercise techniques.

Until now, maybe you've just coasted along in your exercise program without any visible results. Somehow, you look just as soft and untoned as you did a year ago. Have I got news for you!

There are as many as 10 different exercise techniques you can employ to force your body to start burning fat. Some of them have to do with the timing of your workouts, others have to do with special ways to work out. But the common denominator is this: They all represent a surefire approach to getting lean fast. All 10 techniques are covered in Chapter 11 of this book. Don't bypass them!

SECRET #4:
Fuel your fat-burning body.

On the Lean Bodies Workout, you are going to gradually increase the intensity of your workouts, plus perform combination exercise. To do all of this successfully, you've got to have plenty of energy. That energy comes from food. A lot of food! With the Lean Bodies eating program, you gradually increase your calories by 100 to 200 each week — all from specific foods that supercharge your performance and fat-burning potential. (A reminder: Make sure you obtain a copy of my first Lean Bodies book and the *Lean Bodies Cookbook* to learn how my eating program works. Both books are available in paperback.)

"I wish more people would realize how much food you can eat if you make the right choices," says Deb M., who reduced her body fat from 22.4 percent to 15.8 percent by eating approximately 2,000 calories a day on the Lean Bodies program.

You really can't separate nutrition from exercise if your goals are to develop a lean, firm body. Wendy B. found that out early on. She had started weight training 10 years ago in an effort to stave off osteoporosis, which had afflicted her mother. Wendy was also a self-proclaimed aerobics fanatic, attending classes five times a week. The only problem with all this was that she ate a mere two meals a day. After three years of weight training, Wendy had gained only five pounds of muscle. Even though her body fat registered in at a lean 19 percent, she wanted to get leaner still. It's no wonder she wasn't making any progress, considering her extremely sub-par diet.

I persuaded her to try the Lean Bodies eating program, and she was game. I also reduced her aerobic activity to four times a week, for just 30 minutes each session. Here's what Wendy says about her progress:

"The results from the Lean Bodies program of exercise and nutrition were amazing. I gained three pounds of muscle in the first four months. Another four months later, my body fat percentage had dropped to 15.17 percent. Everyone, including my husband, began commenting on my muscles. These compliments gave me the incentive to work out even harder.

"After more than a year on the Lean Bodies program, I decided to compete in a bodybuilding contest. I was at a level that I felt confident enough to get on stage and see how well my physique stacked up.

"Unfortunately, a few months after deciding to compete, I was in a car accident. Thank goodness, only my knee was injured. But

I had to have surgery. I was out of commission for awhile, but I stayed on the Lean Bodies program, adjusting my calories slightly to match my reduced activity level. Sticking with the nutrition program definitely helped me recover more quickly.

"Now at age 50, after seven years of following Cliff's program, I'm a lean 142 1/2 pounds. My energy level is still tremendous, and I have well-defined, beautiful muscles. I feel and look better than I did at age 25. Words cannot express what Cliff and his program have done for me."

SECRET #5:
Develop the mind-set of an athlete.

Many people want to look like a perfectly formed athlete. The Lean Bodies Workout teaches you how to think like an athlete and look like an athlete — but without the grueling schedule of an athlete.

Perhaps up to now you've never considered pushing yourself very far in physical activity because you thought you couldn't. Top athletes refuse to set limits for themselves. The best and often-told example of this is Roger Bannister, the first man to break the four-minute mile. Up until he did it, naysayers said it was humanly impossible to do so. But Bannister did it, and so did four other runners — within only 12 months of Bannister's record. The point is, a lot of what holds us back physically are the mental roadblocks we put up. Adopt an "I can" attitude as you do the Lean Bodies Workout, and you will be amazed at what you can accomplish.

Athletes also chart their performance, their workouts, and their diets by writing everything down. This makes a huge difference in your personal commitment. In a research study I'm conducting, both the experimental groups and the control group are required to write down everything they eat. What I found was that the control group started eating healthier foods, even though they weren't required to do so. Why? Because they had to write it down! Seeing your fitness performance daily in black and white provides a real motivational boost. You'll learn how to chart your own progress, just like an athlete, as part of the Lean Bodies Workout. Easy-to-use charts are included in this book to help you.

Let's Get Moving

Before we jump feet first into the workout, I want to get you "psyched up." What follows are two chapters covering the research-backed benefits of each type of exercise you'll perform on the Lean Bodies Workout. You may already be familiar with some of those benefits. Others will amaze you. Either way, I think they'll provide positive reinforcement as you begin the Lean Bodies Workout.

2

Lean Bodies Aerobics— The Benefits

WHO CAN POSSIBLY KNOW THE BENEFITS of aerobic exercise better than those who do it successfully and get great results?

Take Larry K. His weight had climbed to 350 pounds, with more than 50 percent of it body fat. His heart rate at rest was 95 beats per minute, far too fast but typical for most sedentary people in his condition.

"I started Lean Bodies because I had heard that it was effective, plus a friend had lost more than 40 pounds on it," Larry says. "That convinced me the program was worth a try."

Larry went on to lose body fat by increasing calories and exercising aerobically three to five times a week for 30 to 45 minutes early in the morning.

In the first five weeks on Lean Bodies, he lost 30 pounds and lopped four inches off his waist. Other benefits followed. As Larry tells it: "I have more much energy and endurance than ever, and people comment on how muscular I look."

Larry is also an asthmatic. "I feel the combination of proper eating, weight loss, and aerobic exercise has helped. For instance, my use of my inhaler went from three to four times a day to one to two times a day."

Not only that, Larry's resting heart rate has dropped to 78, an indication that his heart is working more efficiently.

If you don't currently do aerobic exercise, it's time to get with it! As Larry discovered, the benefits are well worth it. Here's a closer look at what aerobic exercise can do for you.

De-Flab Your Body

Aerobic exercise is the best way to lose pure fat — better than dieting alone. At Tufts University, a group of men and women was divided into an exercise group and a diet group. The exercisers worked out twice a day on a stationary bike, burning 360 calories a day but eating the same amount of calories they were consuming before the three-month program started. The dieters were told to cut calories by 360.

At the end of the research period, the dieters lost an average of 11 pounds each. The problem was that six of those pounds were muscle. But the exercisers lost approximately an average of 16 pounds of fat! Even better, they each gained about three pounds of lean muscle.[1]

How exactly does aerobic exercise work its fat-burning potential? You'll learn more about this in Chapter 5, but here's a quick summary: When you exercise aerobically, your body draws on fat in the form of fatty acids as one of its energy sources. Aerobic exercise also increases fat-burning enzymes in your body. You need those enzymes if you want to get lean. Finally, aerobic exercise builds your oxygen-processing capacity. Fat is burned only when there's adequate oxygen around.

Bump Up Your Metabolic Rate

An interesting phenomenon occurs after exercising aerobically. Your metabolic rate (the speed at which your body burns calories) stays elevated after exercise ends. Not only are you burning calories while exercising, you continue to do so later. And the longer you exercise, the longer your metabolic rate stays up.

In one study, five men rode a stationary bicycle at a moderate intensity, randomly varying the length of their rides each day in 30-minute, 45-minute, and 60-minute periods. The researchers found that after the 30-minute ride, the metabolism stayed elevated for 130 minutes; after the 45-minute ride, the metabolism stayed high for 205 minutes. Following the 60-minute ride, the metabolism remained elevated for 455 minutes — the equivalent of an extra 17 minutes of cycling![2]

Where metabolism is concerned, aerobic exercise heats up the metabolic activity of your muscles. Researchers in Japan placed a group of middle-aged women, all slightly overweight, into either an aerobic exercise/diet group or a control group. They wanted to find out what effects aerobic exercise and moderate dietary restriction would have on body composition and metabolism. The women in the exercise/diet group did moderate aerobics from 45 to 60 minutes a day, three to four days a week for 12 weeks.

By the end of the experiment, the exercisers had lost an average of 10 pounds, most of it from fat, but they didn't gain any lean mass. However, the big news was this: The resting metabolic rate per unit of lean mass rose 4 percent. What the study confirms is that while aerobic exercise, combined with moderate dietary restriction, doesn't always increase muscle, it revs up the metabolic activity of the muscle you do have.[3]

By contrast, a sedentary lifestyle lowers your metabolic rate. We've seen evidence of this in studies of patients confined to bed rest whose metabolic rates had plummeted. Even if you're well-trained and well-conditioned, your metabolic rate can drop if you stop exercising for a few days. In studies of highly trained runners who ceased daily training, their metabolic rate dropped by about seven to 10 percent.[4] The lesson here is to stay as active as you can, as much as you can.

Stay Lean Longer

Unless you watch your diet and exercise regularly, you'll naturally put on more body fat as you get older. One main reason is lifestyle. People tend to be less physically active with age. Their muscle mass shrinks, and with it, the ability to efficiently burn calories. Metabolism declines as a result, and it's more difficult for the body to mobilize and burn fat for energy.

But by staying active, you will remain lean. On average, well-trained, middle-aged runners have a body fat percentage of 11 for men and 18 for women,[5] whereas inactive people in the same age group average 27.1 percent for men and 34.4 percent for women.[6] By keeping up your exercise program for as long as you can, you'll postpone unwanted changes in your body composition.

Prevent Heart Disease

The link between aerobic exercise and heart health first came to light in the 1950s. Large-scale studies found that men with sedentary jobs had two times the death rate from heart disease as active workers did.[7]

Since then, many more studies have proved that aerobic exercise is an effective risk-reducer for heart disease. An aerobically trained heart can pump more blood with each beat, during exercise and while at rest. Your heart rate slows, too, so that when you climb a flight of stairs or play a set of tennis, your heart doesn't have to work as hard. You can be more active without running out of breath.

Your entire circulatory system changes, too. Aerobic exercise makes your capillaries increase in size and number, so that more blood finds its way to the muscles and other tissues where it's needed.

Clobber Cholesterol Problems

One important reason aerobic exercise preserves heart health is its positive effect on cholesterol levels. One of the forms of cholesterol in your body is high density lipoprotein cholesterol or HDL. Manufactured mostly in the liver and released into the bloodstream, it appears HDL cholesterol has a protective effect on the heart. It carries other cholesterol away from the arteries and back to the liver so it can be processed. Also, HDL cholesterol removes harmful plaque-causing LDL (low density lipoprotein) cholesterol from the inner walls of arteries feeding the heart. A high level of HDL cholesterol is good for the heart, yet a low level indicates a greater risk for heart disease. These are the reasons HDL cholesterol has earned the nickname "the good cholesterol."

Aerobic exercise plays a big role in raising levels of HDL cholesterol. You can positively change your HDL levels with very little exercise, too — the equivalent of jogging 10 miles a week for nine months. However, if you exercise more intensely as the Lean Bodies Workout recommends, HDL levels can go up even more. In one study, previously inactive men who rode stationary bicycles five times a week for an hour each time at high intensities had an average increase of 13 percent in their HDL cholesterol levels.[8]

Other factors such as diet and family history also play a part in how your cholesterol balances out. But it's clear that exercise is critical. So if you have a cholesterol problem, don't just sit there, exercise!

Reduce High Blood Pressure

High blood pressure, technically known as hypertension, has often been called the "silent killer" because about 60 million Americans have it, but half of them are unaware of it. This can damage your heart, blood vessels, and kidneys, potentially leading to death.

One way to drive blood pressure down is with aerobic exercise. Most studies of hypertensive people show that a reduction can occur with as little as three exercise sessions a week for 30 to 60 minutes each time.

Exercise can prevent high blood pressure, too. A five-year study of 200 hypertension-prone people (aged 30 to 44 years) demonstrated that lifestyle changes, including exercise, could reduce the incidence of high blood pressure. Participants in the study were encouraged to exercise for 30 minutes at least three times a week — and intensely enough to elevate their heart rate to healthy ranges. They chose to do stationary cycling, walking, or swimming. By the end of the study, full-fledged hypertension had occurred in only 8.8 percent of the group.[9] However, be sure to get your doctor's approval before using exercise as a prescription for hypertension.

Stay Energized

While participating in the Lean Bodies classes, Jane S. had to work more than 60 hours two weeks in a row. "It was difficult," she says. "But I know I would have been in worse shape if I hadn't kept doing aerobic exercise five to six times a week. The exercise and the eating program pulled me through the stress of the extra hours."

Ironically, one of the ways to feel more energetic is to expend more energy through aerobic exercise, as Jane discovered.

Aerobic exercise improves your circulation and your respiration — stimulating factors that give you a real lift physically. You're able to do more, with more energy to boot. It's no wonder that so many of our Lean Bodies report that they have energy to spare.

Think Better

With more oxygen traveling to your brain, you think better and more clearly. In a study comparing regular exercisers to inactive people, the exercisers were more decisive and better able to size up a situation.[10]

Also, exercise involving complicated motor skills, such as aerobic dance, affects mental agility, possibly by increasing the amount of oxygen delivered to the brain. Animal studies have found that skill-type exercise creates new brain synapses, special connections that help the brain process more information.

Build Resistance To Disease

Can aerobic exercise be an effective prescription against disease? Quite possibly, according to some recent research. Aerobic exercise appears to bolster your body's army of certain disease-fighting cells. These include:

• Lymphocytes: A type of white blood cell formed in the lymphatic system. About 20 to 30 percent of the white blood cells in the body are lymphocytes. Lymphocytes are responsible for promoting immunity at the cellular level.

• Granulocytes: A white blood cell that is capable of gobbling up harmful invaders.

• Immunoglobulins: An antibody that fights disease-causing microorganisms in the nose and throat.

• Natural killer (NK) cells: A type of lymphocyte that attacks blood-borne viruses.

When you exercise, there's an increase in lymphocytes and granulocytes. In one study, researchers assigned 14 healthy but inactive men, aged 18 to 40, to either an aerobic exercise group or a control group which didn't work out. For 10 weeks, the exercisers trained aerobically three times a week for 45 minutes each time on an exercise bicycle. They exercised at between 70 and 80 percent of their maximum heart rate — a pretty good clip. The important finding of this study was that aerobic training increased several types of lymphocytes.[11]

Also, the harder you work out, the greater the rise in these white blood cells. If your exercise session lasts longer than a half hour, a second increase in white blood cells (mainly granulocytes) occurs, and they stay elevated for up to four hours. This cellular activity suggests that exercise boosts your immunity.

Moderate exercise has an effect on immunoglobulins. In another study, a group of 36 sedentary, mildly obese women participated in a 15-week exercise program of brisk walking five times a week for 45 minutes each time. There was a control group that did not exercise.

At certain intervals during the study, researchers checked the activity of disease-fighting cells in the women's blood, namely lymphocytes and immunoglobulins. Interestingly, moderate exercise did not improve lymphocyte function, but increased the activity of immunoglobulins by 20 percent, especially after only six weeks of training.[12]

In a related study, intense exercise has been shown to increase both the number and activity of NK cells. If the exercise is moderate, however, there's no increase in the number of NK cells. Researchers put 36 sedentary women, ages 25 to 45, on a moderate exercise program to study NK cells. Six weeks of exercise didn't increase NK cell numbers, but it did rev up their activity.[13]

Brighten Up A Blue Mood

Aerobic exercise banishes the blues. That's the conclusion of mounds of studies on aerobic exercise and mental health. In fact, numerous studies have shown that aerobic exercise can be an effective part of treatment for depression and anxiety.[14]

The more you make exercise a habit, the better your mood stays and the lower your stress level, too. But you must make a commitment to it. Researchers in Australia studied three groups of people: long-term exercisers, short-term exercisers, and non-exercisers. The long-term exercisers had a more positive outlook on life and were less stressed out than those in the other two groups, based on the results of questionnaires filled out by the participants.[15]

The Perfect Complement To Aerobic Exercise

I hope all this information is enough to persuade you that aerobic exercise must be incorporated into your exercise lifestyle. Now let's turn to the perfect complement to aerobic exercise — weight training.

3

Lean Bodies Weight Training— The Benefits

WHEN SHE FIRST STARTED LEAN BODIES, Patty E. was not medically cleared to exercise. Nonetheless, she lost 16 pounds in six weeks by gradually increasing her calories to more than 2,000 a day. Soon afterward, Patty got her physician's blessing to begin the Lean Bodies Workout. She started weight training twice a week and performing aerobics three times a week. "Weight training has given me muscle definition and a much more youthful-looking body. In addition, I really do have more strength, particularly in my arms.

"The eating program got my size down to my high school weight; weight training got rid of cellulite and flabby skin."

If you're like many people, you probably have a lot of misconceptions about weight training. Put all of them aside! Weight training is one of the best activities you can adopt for fitness and lifelong health. Let's look at why:

Burn Fat

Most people don't associate weight training with fat-burning. That's a misconception I'll blow out of the water right now! If you want to get leaner, faster, start weight training immediately. Consider the results of a recent study conducted at the University of Maryland: Researchers took 13 healthy men who had never weight trained before and had them lift weights for 16 weeks.

Prior to the program, the researchers checked their body composition with some of the most high-tech measuring techniques available, including magnetic resonance imaging (MRI).

By the end of the 16 weeks, some major changes had occurred. On average, the men lost four pounds of pure fat and gained more than four pounds of lean mass — all because of weight training.[1]

When my wife works out intensely with weights, she feels like she literally forces the fat out of her muscles. Is that possible? It seems so, based on the results of the following study:

A group of women in their 70s started a weight training program in which they worked only their leg muscles. For purposes of comparison, a control group performed endurance-type exercise. Prior to the study, the researchers measured the subjects' body composition — lean mass and body fat — in their legs using high-tech computed tomography (also known as a CT scan).

The weight-trained women boosted their strength levels considerably, compared to the endurance group. Even more interesting was the fact that the weight-trained women showed a decrease in the relative proportion of fat within the quadricep muscle compared with the endurance group. In fact, the researchers noted that fat loss on the endurance-trained women was "negligible."[2] So it appears that you can actually force the fat out!

The message in all of these studies is: Weight training is definitely a fat-burning mode of exercise!

Gain Lean Mass And Muscular Tone

Muscles are like the plants in your house or yard. They wilt and shrivel up not because of old age but because of neglect. With muscle, you use it or lose it!

Weight training makes your muscles develop by causing individual muscle fibers to enlarge (more on this in Chapter 5). This gives your entire body the healthy look of firmness, otherwise known as "muscle tone." Muscle tone basically means that your muscles are a little larger and more defined.

Because of their hormonal makeup, men can develop larger muscles than women can. However, women can achieve comparable strength gains to men who participate in the same weight training program. Weight training also builds muscular endurance — the ability to repeat muscle movements without tiring.

Believe me, it's desirable to build muscle. Developed, toned muscle is what gives your body noticeable shape and definition. You look leaner, fitter, and more youthful when your muscles are weight-trained.

Charge Up Your Metabolism

Strong, toned muscles also are metabolically more active than untoned muscles. In other words, toned muscles burn fat more efficiently, even at rest. That's why it's often said: Muscle is metabolism. The more you have, the more fat you can burn.

Researchers have measured the caloric "afterburn" of weight training — the length of time the metabolic rate is activated following weight training — and have found that it stays elevated for as long as 15 hours afterward![3]

The ability to elevate the metabolic rate is critical, especially if you are starting the Lean Bodies program after a period of restrictive or on-again, off-again dieting. It's no secret that restrictive dieting lowers the metabolic rate, making it hard to lose body fat or build body-toning muscle. Each time you lose then regain fat, muscle tissue is lost, and body fat increases. Since fat burns fewer calories than muscle, it's difficult to control your weight or keep your metabolism running up to speed. The Lean Bodies Workout, combined with nutrition that gradually increases calories from certain types of food, can be just the jump-start your metabolism needs right now.

Get Stronger

Weight training builds strength, which technically means the amount of muscular force you can exert. You need strength for good health and an active life. Strong muscles protect and stabilize your joints and other connective tissues. They help you perform better in sports. A strong body lets you do activities of daily living — carrying groceries, lifting children, mowing the lawn, toting luggage, and so forth — without stress and strain.

You can even do better on your job. When employees performing manual handling jobs at a factory were put on a weight training program, they increased their strength dramatically, as well as their muscular endurance. As a result, the employees felt that they could perform their day-to-day job responsibilities much more easily.[4]

Weight training rebuilds strength even in muscles that have atrophied (shrunk) as a consequence of disease. There's a fascinating story in scientific literature about a woman who had suffered from polio as a child and had chronically and severely weakened muscles as a result. In fact, her condition was getting worse — until she started a weight training program, working out three times a week with five sets of 10 repetitions each workout. Every four months for a year, her strength was tested, and the outcome was remarkable. She increased the muscle strength of her right ankle dorsiflexors by 61 percent and the strength of her left elbow flexors by 32 percent after one year of training. She also started feeling better overall because she was stronger.[5]

Bone Up On Weight Training

Weight training not only develops muscle, it also develops bone mass by stimulating bone cells to produce more bone. This effect has important implications in the prevention of osteoporosis, an age-related disease that results in bone thinning. Women seem to get osteoporosis more often than men — for several reasons. Bone loss in women begins at an earlier age, usually around age 35. Pregnancy and breast-feeding tax stores of bone-building calcium, which is supplied by the skeleton. And women are more likely to go on restrictive diets that are typically low in calcium.

For women, weight training offers an extra measure of protection against osteoporosis. A study at the University of Arizona looked at groups of 40 women, ages 17 to 38. Some were bodybuilders; others were competitive runners; and still others were swimmers and recreational runners. For comparison, a control group was made up of women who did not exercise. When measured, the average bone mineral content of the bodybuilders was consistently denser than that of the runners, swimmers, and controls.[6]

Many other studies of women have turned up similar results. But what about men? Does weight training build men's bones, too? Two studies say — yes.

A group of Swedish scientists studied 40 nationally or internationally ranked male weight lifters to see what effect their physical training had on bone density after their athletic careers were over. Nineteen of the lifters were still working out, and 21 had retired from competition. Bone density in the lifters had been tested in 1975 during their active careers. Fifty-two men matched for age served as a control group for comparison purposes.

The scientists found that bone mass throughout the body (with the exception of the head) was significantly higher in the lifters, compared to the controls. Also, the lifters had the same amount of bone mass in their forearms and knees as they had 15 years ago![7]

The second study I'd like to cite asked this question: What's better for building bone — weight training, running, cross-training (performing a combination of exercise activities), or recreational activities?

A group of active men participated in the study, and the researchers measured their bone content and density using a high-tech body composition measuring method. Body regions measured included the entire skeleton, upper limbs, lower limbs, neck and spine.

Here's what they found: Weight-trained men had the highest bone density in their upper limbs, and runners had the lowest. As for the other body regions, no significant comparisons could be drawn. The researchers concluded that men who regularly weight train have much more bone mass than those who don't.[8]

Keep Your Blood Sugar In Line

With age, we gradually lose the ability to control blood sugar or glucose, putting us at a greater risk of developing Type II diabetes. This is a type of blood sugar metabolism disorder that usually shows up after age 40 in people who are overweight and not physically active and among those with a family history of diabetes. Normally, glucose (blood sugar) gets into cells with the help of the hormone insulin. But in Type II diabetics, the cells aren't sensitive to insulin, probably because there are fewer insulin receptors on the outer cell walls. Glucose, in effect, is barred from entry into cells.

This form of diabetes differs from Type I diabetes, in which not enough insulin is produced. Consequently, muscle, fat, and liver cells can't absorb glucose, which is needed for energy. These patients, who typically get the disease at a young age, must therefore depend on daily injections of the hormone to survive. Type II diabetes doesn't require insulin injections.

All diabetics are at risk for a host of complications, including obesity, eye problems, nerve damage, kidney disease, and cardiovascular disease. Cardiovascular disease, in fact, is the leading cause of death among diabetics.

Studies are showing that maintaining muscle mass, which is sensitive to the body's production of insulin, helps control blood sugar. Weight training helps normalize the flow of glucose from the blood into the muscle tissue where it can be properly used for energy. This effect may help regulate the body's use of glucose, thereby controlling or preventing diabetes and its life-threatening complications.

Build Your Oxygen-Processing Capacity

When you think of oxygen, you usually think lungs. But muscles play a role, too. Muscle is an engine that pushes oxygen throughout the body, including the brain (which uses 20 to 30 percent of the body's oxygen.) The more lean mass you have, the better your body can process oxygen.

Protect Against Cancer

Can lifting weights help prevent cancer? Possibly, since weight training helps whittle away body fat — and excessive body fat is a risk factor for breast and other hormonal-related cancers.

Other types of cancers may be prevented by exercise, too, including colon cancers. In fact, strength training speeds the length of time food spends in the stomach and intestines. Rapid transit through the gastrointestinal tract reduces carcinogenic activity, cutting your risk of developing colon cancer.

There's no concrete proof that weight training and other forms of exercise actually prevent cancer, but the studies conducted thus far point to one conclusion: Physically active people are less likely to get certain types of cancer.

Keep Your Cholesterol In Check

Abnormal levels of blood fats are a risk factor for heart disease and should be checked periodically. There are four measurements usually taken — total blood cholesterol, high density lipoprotein (HDL), low density lipoprotein (LDL), and triglycerides. LDL cholesterol is the harmful kind because it clogs arteries much like lime building up in pipes. This condition eventually leads to atherosclerosis, an accumulation of fatty deposits inside the arteries, which restricts and sometimes cuts off blood flow to vital organs. As noted in the previous chapter, HDL cholesterol works to keep the arteries clear by getting rid of LDL cholesterol.

It's desirable to have a total cholesterol reading of 200 or less. Borderline cholesterol is in the range of 200 to 239, and abnormal cholesterol is 240 or above. One of the factors that can lower and normalize your cholesterol — in addition to a low-fat, high-fiber diet — is exercise. For a long time, scientists have known that aerobic exercise was an effective cholesterol-fighter. But now there's overwhelming scientific proof that weight training can dramatically lower the level of fats in your blood.

In one study, cholesterol and triglyceride levels dropped significantly in men and women who weight trained for 16 weeks. The women reduced their LDL cholesterol by nearly 18 percent, and their triglycerides by 28.3 percent. The men were just as successful, particularly in cutting their LDL cholesterol (by 16.2 percent). [9]

In another study, 11 healthy, untrained men ages 44 to 55 were studied to see what effects a 16-week program of weight training would have on certain risk factors for heart disease, including cholesterol, glucose levels, and blood pressure. For comparison purposes, there was a sedentary control group used in the study.

By the end of the study, the training program had produced, on average, a 13 percent increase in HDL cholesterol (the protective kind), a 5 percent reduction in low-density cholesterol (the harmful variety), and an 8 percent decrease in total cholesterol. The weight-trained men were able to tolerate a glucose feeding better — an indication that their muscle cells were probably handling glucose efficiently. What's more, the subjects' blood pressure was reduced. These findings led the researchers to conclude that weight training is a definite plus when it comes to lowering risk factors for heart disease. [10]

Postpone The Effects Of Aging

The loss of muscle tone and strength is a process that begins in your late twenties — unless you undertake a regular exercise program that includes weight training. Weight training is the only exercise known to regenerate vital body tissue (muscle), regardless of age. In one recent study, 20 people aged 51 to 81 participated in a

12-week weight training program to see if they could build lean mass and strength. On average, the men upped their strength by more than 66 percent; the women, by more than 72 percent.[11]

This is just one of hundreds of studies popping up, all with the same conclusion: You are never too old to start pumping iron!

The Next Step

If you recall, secret #1 for burning body fat is to gradually increase your intensity in both weight training and aerobic exercise. That's the first order of business for getting lean fast — and the topic we'll cover in the next chapter.

4

The Intensity Factor In Fat-Burning

PRIOR TO STARTING the Lean Bodies Workout and eating program, Debbie K. was toting around 28 per-cent body fat, a lot for a woman. Around mid-day, her energy levels would nosedive, and she'd head to the bedroom for a nap, probably because she was using a milkshake-type diet in an effort to control her weight. Clearly, it wasn't working.

So Debbie came to Lean Bodies and began the pro-gram. Before long, she had doubled her daily caloric intake and started exercising as hard as any athlete. Her body fat percentage dropped to a lean 18 percent, and she no longer had to take naps. What's more, she began feeling stronger and looking more defined.

As Debbie puts it: "Since starting the program, I have increased my stamina so I can exercise longer and harder. I can now maintain my heart rate at a higher level (165 to 170), even for a full hour. I weight train three times a week, perform aero-bics five times a week, and play racquetball once or twice a week — all with energy to spare!"

Wouldn't you like to be a powerhouse like Debbie? You can be, as long as you increase your calories, get active, and begin to gradually increase your exercise intensity — secret #1 in burning body fat. Intensity simply means pushing yourself and continually striving to reach the next level.

Is that hard? No, as long as you're fueling your body with ample calories and nutrients. Is that fun or is it work? It's fun! Especially when you start reaping the rewards: a lean, firm body, more energy, even a slowdown in some of the physical signs of aging. Not to mention the compliments you'll get from people.

I want you to set your mind and body in high-gear as we look at exactly what intensity is, and what it can do for you. There are two types of intensity: aerobic intensity and weight training intensity.

Aerobic Intensity

Aerobic intensity refers to how hard you work out when you're walking, jogging, running, bicycling, swimming, or performing any other type of heart-pumping activity. To burn fat and build cardiovascular health, you must gradually increase the intensity of your exercise effort. Aerobic intensity is generally described in one of two ways: VO_2 max and heart rate.

VO_2 Max

VO_2 max, otherwise known as "aerobic capacity," describes the ability of your body to take in, transport, and use oxygen. It is usually expressed as a percentage of "oxygen consumption" during exercise, or put another way, the maximum amount of oxygen you use while working out aerobically. A usage of 40 to 60 percent of VO_2 max is considered moderate intensity; more than 60 percent of VO_2 max is considered vigorous or high intensity. If you've never exercised much in the past and you start an aerobic exercise program, you can increase your VO_2 max by up to 20 percent by working out at a good clip at least three times a week.[1] VO_2 max stays higher in people who exercise aerobically.

Is there a way to tell what your VO_2 max is while exercising? Exact VO_2 max is measured in laboratory settings with special devices and techniques, so unless you have access to a lab, you can't really get a specific percentage for your aerobic capacity. However, a good rule of thumb to follow is this: If you're breathing hard, yet still able to carry on a conversation, you're working out in the higher-intensity range of your VO_2 max. When you exercise in this range, more oxygen can be "extracted" by your muscles, and more stored fat and carbohydrate can be used to supply energy.

Heart Rate

Heart rate indicates the amount of work your heart does to keep up with the demands of various activities, including exercise. At rest, your heart averages 60 to 80 beats a minute. This is referred to as your "resting heart rate." In unexercised, sedentary people, the resting heart rate can be as high as 100 beats per minute or more. By contrast, well-trained endurance athletes may have resting heart rates in the range of 28 to 40 beats a minute.[2] The more fit you become aerobically, the lower your resting heart rate becomes.

During exercise, your heart rate increases in direct proportion to your exercise effort. The rate at which your heart beats during exercise is called "exercising heart rate."

For best results, you should exercise at a level sufficient enough to raise your heart rate to 70 to 85 percent or higher of your maximum heart rate (MHR). MHR is expressed as 220 minus your age. For example, suppose you're 35 years old, and you start an aerobic exercise program. Your maximum heart rate is 185 (220 - 35). You should work out at an intensity such that your heart reaches between 130 and 157 beats a minute (85 percent of 185 beats per minute = .85 x 185 = 157).

If you are not exercising now, start working out in the lower end of your range for at least 30 minutes. Gradually increase your intensity so that you reach the higher end of your range as your body becomes more aerobically conditioned. Also, the better conditioned you become, the greater ability you have to exceed the 85 percent range. Always strive for higher intensities as safely as you can sustain them.

Use the chart in Table 4-1 to identify your target heart training range, based on your age.

Your Target Heart Training Range

Age	*Beats Per Minute*
20	140 - 170
25	137 - 166
30	133 - 162
35	130 - 157
40	126 - 153
45	123 - 149
50	119 - 145
55	116 - 140
60	112 - 136
65	109 - 132
70	105 - 128

Table 4-1

How to Obtain Your Heart Rate
During Aerobic Exercise

There are four methods to determine your heart rate while exercising:

- Finger on carotid artery (Dont press hard).
- By placing your hand directly over your heart at the left breast.
- By placing your finger at the radial artery on your wrist.
- At the temporal artery at the front of the ear.

So stick to one of the three recommended methods for calculating your heart rate. To find your heart rate per minute, simply count the beats for 10 seconds and multiply by six.

Keep records of both your resting heart rate and your heart rate during exercise. This information will help you evaluate your progress on the Lean Bodies Workout. Your resting heart rate (your heart rate in the morning before you get out of bed) should decrease over time. If not, or if your resting heart rate suddenly jumps up to a higher level, this could signal a medical problem, and you should check it out with your physician.

Other Factors Influencing Aerobic Intensity

To reap the benefits of aerobic exercise, from fat-burning to cardiovascular strengthening, you have to go beyond a certain minimum requirement for positive changes to occur. We've just looked at this from the perspective of intensity. In addition, there are two other intensity-related ways to increase your exercise effort: exercise duration and exercise frequency.

Exercise Duration

Exercise duration refers to the length of time you work out. As the duration of your exercise increases, you start burning more fat for fuel. On the Lean Bodies Workout, gradually build up to exercising aerobically for 30 to 45 minutes or longer each session to maximize your fat-burning potential. At the same time, you should work on increasing your aerobic intensity.

Exercise Frequency

Research shows that you derive the best aerobic benefits from working out three to five times week. A word of caution: Newcomers to aerobic exercise should not start out exercising five times a week! If you do, you will risk burnout. Instead, start out by trying to exercise three times a week, then gradually build to five sessions as your aerobic capacity improves or as your personal schedule permits.

The Value of Increasing Duration and Frequency

A simple increase in the duration and frequency of your aerobic exercise can make a tremendous difference in your progress. Take the case of Brad R. Brad had gone up and down in weight for many years, usually due to yo-yo dieting and poor nutritional practices. At his highest weight, he tipped the scales at 320 pounds.

Brad started Lean Bodies in 1995 and increased his calories as recommended. He upped the frequency and duration of his aerobic exercise, too. Where once he walked, he now started running—as much as three to five miles each time. Gradually Brad increased his workouts from two to three times a week to three to four times a week. The result? Today Brad has stripped down to 228 pounds, with a body fat percentage of 17.2. According to his body composition measurements, Brad has gained 9 pounds of lean muscle and has peeled away 15 pounds of pure fat.

How Important Is Aerobic Exercise Intensity?

I believe the issue of intensity has been underplayed in the past. Research indicates overwhelmingly that higher-intensity exercise produces greater fitness benefits than less intense activity. Here are some examples of studies showing that milder-intensity activities don't make much of an impact on body fat:

• In a study at the Loma Linda University School of Nutrition, overweight women were randomly assigned to either an exercise group or a non-exercise group. Those in the exercise group walked briskly five times a week for 45 minutes for 15 weeks. The findings were not what you would assume: The exercising women lost no weight. Nor was there much positive change in health factors such as cholesterol and triglyceride levels. The researchers concluded that moderate exercise wasn't enough of a stimulus to change body composition or blood fats in overweight women. [4]

• Another study looked into the effects of brisk walking on body fat, body fat distribution, and endurance in a group of women. Twenty-eight of these women, who prior to the study had been sedentary, were asked to follow a walking program for a year, and 16 women served as a control group. On average, the walkers logged in 157 minutes a week of brisk walking over the year.

By the end of the study, the bad news was that brisk walking didn't produce any significant changes in body fat percentage or body fat distribution. But the good news was that exercise improved endurance and lowered heart rate. [5]

Now before we draw any conclusions from these studies, I don't want you to get the idea that brisk walking is a waste of time. For people beginning an exercise program, it's the best possible starting point. We love walking as an aerobic choice on the Lean Bodies Workout, especially for beginning exercisers! Just build your walking speed! For more active people, the message in these studies is that it's beneficial to push a little harder. Of course, you should be cleared by your physician before increasing intensity.

Now let's switch gears for a moment by looking at what higher-intensity exercise can achieve:

• In a study of Harvard alumni, researchers noted a 39 percent reduction in cardiovascular disease risk factors among those who exercised at higher intensities.[6]

• From surveys and medical records of 6,849 male runners with an average age of 45, researchers in California discovered that cardiovascular benefits, mainly better cholesterol profiles, improved with exercise intensity. Runners who logged the most miles per week had the highest HDL cholesterol, the lowest total cholesterol, the lowest triglycerides, and healthier body-weights overall.[7]

• A group of Canadian researchers evaluated 1,366 women and 1,257 men to see what effect exercise intensity had on body fat and body fat distribution. The researchers evaluated the subjects' aerobic capacity, checked their body fat by taking skinfold measurements, and took body circumference measurements. Next, the subjects were placed into one of four groups, based on the type of exercise they did. Interestingly, those who participated in the most vigorous activities on a regular basis had lower body fat percentages and smaller body dimensions than those not performing such intense activities.[8]

Weight Training Intensity

Intensity in weight training refers primarily to the demand you place on your muscles — in other words, how much weight you can lift. Intensity is ever-changing. What felt heavy to you last week may feel lighter this week because your muscles are responding to the demands placed on them and growing stronger as a result.

Progressive Overload

"Progressive overload" is a key factor in weight training intensity. For your muscles to respond — that is, get stronger and better developed — you have to "overload" them. That means continually putting more demands on them than they're used to — in other words, increasing your weight training intensity.

Muscles adapt to greater and greater demands. For example, let's say all you can lift on the arm curl right now is 40 pounds. But a few workouts later that same 40 pounds feels light. Your muscles have adapted to 40 pounds. You are now ready to challenge your arm muscles with 45 pounds. Once the muscles have adapted to that demand, you can bump the weight up again.

You should gradually increase your poundages on all exercises in the Lean Bodies Workout as your muscles get used to certain poundages. The trick is to keep pushing yourself each workout and gradually crank up the difficulty level. Overloading the muscles in this manner activates muscle fibers so that they get stronger, more toned, and better developed. This all adds up to more fat-burning power.

Another factor that plays a part in weight training intensity is the number of repetitions you do on a given exercise. Sometimes, it's difficult to increase a poundage. Until you can, it's best to increase the number of times (repetitions) you lift that weight.

There are other intensity-builders you can use as you advance in your weight training program. You'll learn more about them in Chapter 12.

Turn Intensity Into Results

When you put into practice the concepts of intensity discussed here, some amazing things happen inside your body. In the next chapter, you will learn what goes on inside to produce the positive changes taking place on the outside.

5

CHAPTER FIVE

How Your Body Responds To The Lean Bodies Workout

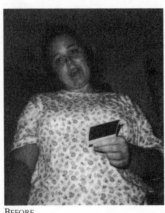

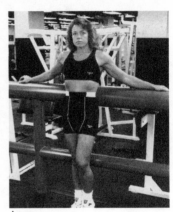

BEFORE   AFTER

"I WAS A REAL COUCH POTATO before starting the Lean Bodies Workout and eating program!" says Lynn C., above. "I was always sluggish, tired, with no energy. Worse, I weighed 180 pounds, and my body fat measurement was 37 percent."

Lynn chose Lean Bodies because "it seemed to be a program I could incorporate into my daily lifestyle for the rest of my life."

So Lynn went to work, gradually increasing her calories from wholesome foods, exercising, and increasing the intensity of her workouts. She mastered all the principles of Lean Bodies while attending our classes in Dallas.

Seven months later, she walked up to me at a gym, and I didn't even recognize her

Lynn gradually built up to working out aerobically six times a week (running, step aerobics, treadmill walking, and stairclimbing on a machine), plus weight training three times a week. Here's what she has to say about the results of increasing her intensity:

"When I began the Workout, I hired a personal trainer. In the beginning, I whined a lot. He wouldn't put up with it; eventually, neither would I. Now, if I don't work out super-hard, I feel like I haven't done a good workout. The harder, the better. As a result, I have really lean muscle striations in my arms and legs. I didn't know those muscles existed!

"I'm stronger now than I've ever been. I continually get looks from people. I can't function without my aerobic exercise, either. It refreshes me, clears my mind, relieves stress, and keeps body fat off. Prior to Lean Bodies, my self-esteem had hit rock bottom. Now I have confidence and carry myself very well."

Throughout the seven-month period of doing Lean Bodies, Lynn had her body fat regularly checked using skinfold caliper measurements (this system is explained in the next chapter). Her numbers are inspiring! From a weight of 187, Lynn now weighs 136 pounds; from a body fat percentage of 37, she now measures a lean, firm 13 percent. Furthermore, she scaled 11 inches off her waist!

It Can Happen To You, Too

The same remarkable changes experienced by Lynn can take place with your body, too, when you follow the Lean Bodies Workout and eating program. You will begin to see changes in the way you look and feel, at rest and during exercise — in just a few short weeks. You might notice that you are getting stronger or that you feel less winded climbing a flight of stairs. It seems like your heart is beating more slowly while you are at your desk or watching television. You begin to see more muscle definition on your body, and formerly too-tight clothes now fit. You have more energy from morning to bedtime. All in all, your body feels like it's in a healthy sync. These positive changes as a result of regular exercise are technically known as "adaptations to exercise." Your body is making these changes to help it respond better to exercise. Let's take a look at exactly what's going on inside your body to produce these wonderful "adaptations."

Energy Production

To breathe, exercise, or perform any type of activity, your body requires energy from food. In a series of biochemical reactions, the nutrients from food are broken into a form of chemical energy that powers your every move. This food-to-fuel process is collectively known as metabolism. Metabolism creates the energy required for sustaining life.

Energy is produced in the cell, the smallest component in your body. With the exception of the human egg cell, cells can be seen only with the help of a microscope. There are many different types of cells in the body, and they come in all shapes and sizes.

One of the basic functions of a cell is to take nutrients and turn them into forms that can be used by the body for energy. Inside the cell is a structure called a mitochondrion, a site where all energy-producing reactions take place. Mitochondria are often referred to as the "energy factories" of cells.

Of interest to exercisers is the muscle cell, which is actually a muscle fiber. Muscles are made up of hundreds of these tiny threadlike fibers. Muscle fibers, like all cells, run on a high-energy compound known as ATP (adenosine triphosphate). This is a molecular fuel that makes muscles contract, conducts nerve impulses, and promotes other cellular energy processes. ATP is made naturally by muscle cells from mixing oxygen with the nutrients in the food you eat.

Sources Of Energy

Energy from food comes from the breakdown of carbohydrate, fat, and, to some extent, protein. Carbohydrate is one of the main sources of energy for exercise. During digestion, carbohydrate is broken down into glucose, also known as blood sugar. Glucose is stored in the muscles and liver as glycogen until your cells are ready to convert it into ATP.

During this conversion, stored glycogen is broken down back into glucose, then carried by your blood to the exercising muscles to be metabolized for energy. Glycogen reserves are limited and can be emptied if not replaced by dietary carbohydrate. Some glucose circulates naturally in the blood, and this is used for energy, too.

The other major energy store in your body is fat. In fact, it's the largest reservoir of stored energy on your body. Fats are stored primarily as triglycerides in fat tissues and muscles, but also as free fatty acids (FFAs) in the blood. It has been estimated that an average man could cycle 2,000 miles if his stored body fat were converted to muscular energy.[1]

With so much fat packed away, why not burn it instead of glycogen? Fat is harder to break down than glycogen. To be metabolized, fat requires the presence of oxygen — unlike glycogen, which can be burned with or without oxygen. The Lean Bodies Workout will show you ways to mobilize body fat stores more rapidly for use as fuel.

Protein's primary job is to build and repair body tissues. During metabolism, it is broken down into sub-units called amino acids. Under certain exercise conditions, amino acids are pressed into service to yield energy. Both protein and fat can be converted into glucose, if needed.

The Three Energy Systems Of The Body

Your cells generate ATP through one of three energy systems: the phosphagen system, the glycolytic system, and the oxidative system.

The job of the phosphagen system is to rebuild ATP by supplying a compound called creatine phosphate or CP. Once ATP is used up, it must be replenished by additional food and oxygen. During short bursts of exercise, like weight training or sprinting, there isn't sufficient oxygen available to the working muscles. At that point, CP kicks in. It can supply energy for a few short seconds of work. CP can help create ATP when ATP is used up.

Any intense exercise lasting for three to 15 seconds will rapidly deplete ATP and CP in a muscle. Beyond that point, they must then be replaced. Replenishing ATP and CP is the job of the other energy systems in the body.

The glycolytic system makes more glucose available to the muscles, either from the breakdown of dietary carbohydrates during digestion or from the breakdown of muscle and liver glycogen. In a process called glycolosis, glycogen is dismantled into glucose in the muscles through a series of chemical reactions to ultimately form more ATP.

Several hormones are involved in this process. The catecholamines, norepinephrine and epinephrine (also known as adrenaline), trigger the breakdown of muscle glycogen into glucose for use by muscle cells. Similarly, the hormone glucagon promotes the conversion of liver glycogen into glucose. During exercise, there's a rise in glucagon. Cortisol levels also increase during exercise. This hormone frees up amino acids to be used in the liver to produce glucose. Once glucose gets to the muscle cells, the hormone insulin lets it gain entry.

The glycogen stockpiled in your muscles can supply enough energy for about two to three minutes of short-burst exercise at a time. If there's abundant oxygen available to the muscle cell, a lot of ATP will be made. If oxygen is absent or in short supply, then the muscles will produce a waste product called lactic acid from glucose. A buildup of lactic acid in a working muscle creates a burning sensation and causes the muscle to stop contracting. Removal of lactic acid requires oxygen to burn food to replenish CP and ATP. A brief rest period gives the body time to deliver oxygen to the muscles, and you can continue exercising.

The third energy system in your body is the oxidative system. It is called into play for aerobic exercise and other endurance activities. Although the oxygen system can handle the energy needs of endurance exercise, all three energy systems kick in to some degree. The phosphagen and glycolytic energy systems dominate when you are weight training.

Oxygen isn't used as a direct source of energy for exercise, only as an ingredient to produce large amounts of ATP from other energy sources. The oxygen system works as follows: You breathe in oxygen, which is subsequently taken up by your lungs. Your heart pumps oxygen-rich blood to tissues, including muscle. Inside muscle cells, the mitochondria turn carbohydrates and fats into energy through a series of energy-producing reactions.

How Your Body Burns Fat During Exercise

At mild exercise intensities — below 50 percent of VO_2 max — about half your total energy comes from stored carbohydrate (glycogen) and the other half comes from fat. As intensity and duration increase, more carbohydrate and fat are used for fuel. After about an hour or more of very intense exercise, your glycogen stores get low, and your body starts drawing primarily on fat for energy.

Is there a way to get the body to tap into fat stores earlier? You bet. In Chapter 11, there are several techniques you can use to activate your fat stores.

The major fat sources used during exercise are free fatty acids in the blood and "triglycerides," a storage form of fat in the muscle and in fat tissues. There's such a low reserve of blood-borne free fatty acids, however, that they must be replenished by the huge stores of triglycerides packed away in the body.

Getting these triglycerides out of storage is the job of several hormones. They are cortisol; the catecholamines, adrenaline (epinephrine) and norepinephrine; and growth hormone. The first to go to work is cortisol. It helps release fatty acids into the blood so they can be taken up in the cells and burned for energy. After 30 to 45 minutes of exercise, levels of cortisol peak, then return to normal. At that point, other hormones take over the cortisol's job.

The hormones norepinephrine and epinephrine trigger the breakdown of triglycerides to fatty acids inside fat cells. Muscle triglycerides are also broken down to produce fatty acids. The fatty acids cross the cell membrane to the blood and are transported to muscle cells. There, they enter the mitochondria and undergo a series of complex reactions to produce energy through the oxygen energy system.

Growth hormone is released during and just after intense exercise. It mobilizes fat from storage and makes more fat available for energy. Growth hormone also promotes the transport of certain essential amino acids inside muscle cells to stimulate muscle growth. For these reasons, growth hormone is one of the most important hormones for exercisers because of its powerful actions in fat-burning and muscle-building.

Changes Inside Muscle Cells
As A Result Of Aerobic Exercise

Some remarkable things are happening at the level of the muscle cell as you become more aerobically fit. For example:

• There's an increase in a substance called myoglobin. Myoglobin stores oxygen and helps escort it from the bloodstream to the mitochondria during exercise. The higher your myoglobin supply, the better your aerobic endurance.

• Mitochondria increase in size and number. This means your cells are capable of burning nutrients, including fat, more efficiently.

• Your muscle fibers develop a greater capacity to build up and store fat-burning enzymes — special chemicals that encourage your muscle fibers to burn fat for energy. In short, your muscle fibers are now capable of using up more fat. These changes can take place in the first eight weeks of working out.

• Aerobic exercise increases your VO_2 max (your aerobic capacity), and this in turn enhances the ability of your muscles to better combust fat as fuel. At the cellular level, the breakdown of triglycerides speeds up, and they're released faster from fat cells. So the better trained you are aerobically, the better your body can burn fat. Highly conditioned runners can draw as much as 75 percent of their fuel from fat even while running at about 70 percent of their VO_2 max.

• Your muscle fibers have the ability to store more glycogen. That means you have a better supply of glycogen for energy. With more stored glycogen, you can work out harder, at higher intensities, and achieve even better results.

Other Important Changes In Muscle Fibers

Some other things are happening, too: Certain muscle fibers undergo important changes in composition. Your muscle is composed of two types of muscle fibers: slow-twitch fibers and fast-twitch fibers. Slow-twitch fibers, also known as Type I, contract at a relatively slow speed, compared to the fast-twitch variety, and are used for endurance-type exercises such as long distance running. Of all muscle fibers, the slow-twitch variety have the most mitochondria in them. Slow-twitch fibers burn fat for energy.

Fast-twitch fibers contract quickly and are called into play during strength and power activities. There are two types of fast-twitch fibers, Type IIa and Type IIb. Type IIa fibers can burn fat for energy to power muscular contractions, whereas Type IIb uses glycogen. Type IIa fibers contain more mitochondria than Type IIb, but fewer than that found in Type I fibers.

Long-duration, high-intensity aerobics and high-intensity weight training, as recommended on the Lean Bodies Workout, increase the total number of mitochondria in fast-twitch fibers to levels higher than those found in slow-twitch muscle fibers. By increasing mitochondria inside these muscle fibers, you turn your muscles into super fat-burners.

Channels To The Muscles

With any type of endurance training, the number of capillaries surrounding each muscle fiber increases. Capillaries are the smallest branches of blood vessels, and their job is to channel nutrients to cells and take waste products away. The more capillaries you have, the better your muscle fibers are fed with nutrients for growth and repair. The build-up of muscle capillaries can take place rapidly — within just a few weeks of training. With longer periods of training, capillaries can increase by as much as 15 percent.[2]

Exercise Shrinks Fat Cells

With exercise, changes occur in fat cells, too. They actually shrink, resulting in a smaller fat cell. But if you stop working out, fat cells get larger, something that can happen quickly.[3]

Changes In Your Heart As A Result Of Aerobic Exercise

Aerobic exercise makes your heart muscle pump with greater force. As the heart works harder, it becomes stronger. It does so by increasing in size, causing several positive adaptations:

• Your heart can pump more blood with every beat.

• Your heart can recover faster after exercise.

• You gain a lower resting heart rate.

• There's greater blood flow to exercising muscles, therefore more oxygen is available.

Taken together, these changes and those occurring inside and around muscle fibers greatly enhance your exercise performance and overall health.

Changes In Muscle Cells As A Result Of Weight Training

There are three types of muscle in your body: skeletal muscle, which is used for movement of the skeleton; smooth muscle, which lines internal organs and intestines; and heart muscle. They all work the same way — by contracting and relaxing. This is possible because the fibers that make up muscles can shorten their length by 30 to 40 percent.

Skeletal muscles represent the largest soft tissue mass in your body, comprising some 660 muscles and about 15 to 40 percent of your weight, depending on your muscular fitness. They contract when stimulated by nerve impulses and relax when the impulse is gone.

The smooth muscles and the heart muscle aren't under such control, but have their own mechanisms and contract without needing instructions from nerve impulses.

The muscle of interest to exercisers is skeletal muscle. Skeletal muscles get larger and firmer because of the effect exercise has on muscle fibers. Technically, muscle growth is known as *muscle hypertrophy* — which means that an individual muscle fiber gets bigger as structural changes take place inside it. If you examine a skeletal muscle fiber under a microscope, you'll see that it's made up of many sub-units called *fibrils*. These are constructed of long filaments of *actin* and *myosin*, two types of *contractile protein*. They can slide over each other like two pieces of a telescope to cause contraction. When you build muscle, you are essentially increasing the amount of contractile proteins in your muscle fibers. This makes the muscle fibers increase in diameter, get stronger, and generate more force when they contract.

Exercise causes microscopic tears in your muscles. By lifting a weight, you force the muscle to lengthen when it wants to contract. This literally tears apart the tiny structures of the muscle (the cause of the muscle soreness you feel 24 to 48 hours after a workout). Inflammation sets in, and immune system cells rush to the scene to repair the damage. The tissues are restored in the process. But an interesting phenomenon takes place: The body makes the muscle fibers bigger and stronger to protect itself against future trauma.

The building material for this growth and repair process comes primarily from protein, broken down in digestion into amino acids. They enter the bloodstream and are transported to cells to be re-synthesized into body proteins. Muscle cells use amino acids to create more actin and myosin.

Although most research proves that muscle growth is a result of hypertrophy, there's some evidence that muscle grows by *hyperplasia*, the addition of more muscle fibers. Studies demonstrating hyperplasia have been done mostly with animals, and the results are intriguing. In one study, cats flexed their right wrists against increasing resistance over a period of 101 weeks. When scientists compared the muscle fibers of the right wrists to the left wrists, they found 9 percent more fibers in the exercised muscles.[4] But we need more work with human subjects to see if the body can really make new muscle fibers.

Changes In Bone And Connective Tissue

Exercise builds bone and connective tissue, too. When you place stress on your bones with activity such as weight training, more bone-strengthening minerals (including calcium) are deposited within them. Consequently, bone width and bone thickness both increase, and your bones get stronger. Although the exact mechanism hasn't been identified, connective tissues such as joints, ligaments, and tendons get stronger and denser, too, as a result of exercise.

An Amazing Machine

There's no doubt about it, your body is an amazing machine. And you are the operator with the ability to fine-tune it to perfection with the right kind of exercise and nutrition.

6

Getting Started

BY NOW, I HOPE YOU'RE READY to take action —
that is, start the Lean Bodies Workout. Before you do,
however, it's wise to get a medical evaluation first, and
along with it, a body composition analysis. Knowing
where you stand medically and physically helps you
work out more safely and effectively, plus motivates you
to change your current fitness level.

Your Pre-Participation Examination

Always check with your physician before beginning
any type of exercise program. In fact, it may be wise for you to
undergo a thorough examination as well as exercise testing, particularly if you're a healthy man over 40, a healthy woman over
50, or have any risk factors for heart disease, such as a family history of heart disease, high blood pressure, or high cholesterol.
Naturally, if you have symptoms of any illness or lingering
injuries, you must be checked out thoroughly and given the okay
of your physician prior to starting an exercise program.[1]

The purpose of such an examination is to determine your general health, identify any conditions that might limit your partici-
pation, and detect any cardiovascular, respiratory, neurological, or
muscular problems and their severity. The exam may involve mul-
tiple tests. One might be a questionnaire on your medical history
on which you'll be asked to answer questions regarding your over-

all health, past hospitalizations and surgeries, diseases, allergies, medication use, and family history of illnesses.

A physical exam may evaluate the health status of your heart, chest, and lungs; the strength of various body parts; orthopedic status; the condition of other body parts and organs; and your percentage of body fat. A blood test also might be administered to determine cholesterol levels. Depending on your age, you may also undergo treadmill testing to detect any cardiovascular irregularities. Identifying any type of abnormality — or simply verifying that you're fit — can make you a more effective exerciser and a healthier person overall.

An Easy Way To Test Your Body Composition

The most valid method of measuring body fat and lean muscle is body composition testing. Essentially, body composition refers to how much body fat and lean muscle you have and is expressed in percentages. This assessment is more important than just knowing your weight on the scales. Weight is bones, muscle, fat, and water taken together in one lump measurement.

Checking yourself against weight-and-height charts, for example, isn't such a good idea, since it can be very misleading. These charts don't tell you much about the composition of your body. If you are a man who weighs 200 pounds, for instance, yet is only 10 percent body fat, you might be considered overweight according to the charts, when in fact, you are quite lean and fit. Charts lead you to believe that you weigh too much. However, that extra weight might be lean tissue — exactly what you want.

Your body composition test provides the benchmark against which you'll measure your progress. At the end of the eight weeks, your body fat percentage will be lower, and your lean muscle will be higher. This positive shift in body composition will only affirm what you see in the mirror — a leaner, firmer you.

There are many methods of assessing body composition — underwater weighing, ultrasound, electrical impedance, and computerized tomography (CT scans), to name just a few. None of these methods is 100 percent accurate; all have certain limitations. However, one of the best and most convenient methods is the skinfold caliper. Besides being very accurate, it is inexpensive, and the measurements can be taken quickly.

The caliper is a special instrument that measures the amount of fat just under the skin. With this instrument, you take measurements at various points on the body and plug them into a formula that converts the measurement to body fat and lean muscle percentages. You can purchase a skinfold caliper device from pharmacies, gyms, health food stores, and fitness mail order companies. Many gyms and health clubs perform skinfold caliper assessments as a service for their members. If you would like to have a skinfold caliper device for home use, ordering information is located in Appendix C.

How To Take Skinfold Measurements

Here are some guidelines to follow to ensure the accuracy of this technique:

1. A person experienced in using the caliper should perform the measurements. Ideally, you should have the same person measure your skinfolds each time you need to check your body fat.

2. The measurer should grasp the skinfold by thumb and index finger about two inches apart and pull it away from the body. The amount pinched should be enough to make a fold with parallel sides.

3. The caliper can be held in either hand, perpendicular to the skinfold, with the instrument scale facing up.

4. The measurer should place the jaw of the caliper on the skinfold in a position that's neither too deep nor too close to the top of the skinfold.

5. The measurer next releases the trigger so that the entire force of the jaws is on the skinfold. Keep the skinfold elevated with the fingers of your left hand, without releasing pressure.

6. Several seconds later, the scale can be read. The reading should then be recorded.

7. For accuracy, take at least two readings at each site.

8. Don't take measurements when the skin is wet, since this causes too much skin to be pinched. Nor should measurements be taken immediately after exercise. There's a movement of body fluid to the skin at this time, and this causes an inaccurate reading.

How To Measure

You can measure skinfolds at either five or nine sites on the body. The five-point system is an easy way to determine your body fat percentage; the nine-point system also is an easy way. Here's how to measure your body fat percentage using the five-point system.

The Five-Point System

1. Triceps. The measurer should take the measurement at the bottom of the inside triceps head, using a vertical skinfold.

2. Abdominals. Measure a vertical fold one inch to the right or left side of and one inch below the navel.

3. Iliac crest. The ilium is the upper and largest of the three bones of that compose either lateral half of the pelvis. The crest

portion of the ilium is the top rounded portion of the lateral half of the pelvis, just over the hip and in the middle of the body.

4. Subscapular. This site is located on the back. Find the bottom of the shoulder blade, then move one inch in toward the spine. The measurer should pull the skinfold in a vertical direction.

5. Measure a vertical fold in the center of the thigh, midway between the kneecap and the hip.

After measuring these sites, plug the numbers into the following formula and use the worksheet in Table 6-1 to help you.

1. Figure your bodyweight in kilograms: Bodyweight in pounds divided by 2.2 = BW.

2. Multiply your height in inches by .254 = Ht.

3. $\sqrt{(\frac{BW}{Ht.})} \times 3 \times .741$ = Variable

4. Add the five skinfold measurements.

5. $\frac{\text{Sum of Skinfold}}{\text{Variables}}$ = Bodyfat%

Body Composition Worksheet — Five-Point System

Name: _____

Date: _____ Weight: _____

Measurements

Triceps _____	Subscapular _____
Adominals _____	Thigh _____
Iliac Crest _____	

Calculations

- Bodyweight in kilograms = _____
  (bodyweight divided by 2.2)
- Height in inches x .254 = _____
- Variable = _____
  (bodyweight in kg divided by height x .254)
- Total Skinfolds = _____
- Body Fat Percentage = _____
  (sum of skinfolds divided by variable)

Table 6-1

The Nine-Point System

1. Chest. Measure about one inch below the collarbone and three to four inches from the inside of the chest muscle. With women, make sure the measurement is not on breast tissue. The skinfold should be pulled in a horizontal direction.

2. Subscapular. This site is located on the back. Find the middle of the shoulder blade, then move one inch in toward the spine. The measurer should pull the skinfold in a vertical direction.

3. Biceps. The measurement is taken in the middle of the biceps, with the skinfold pulled in a vertical direction.

4. Triceps. The measurer should take the measurement at the bottom of the inside triceps head, using a vertical skinfold.

5. Kidney. Find the dimple just above your buttocks. Move up two inches and out two inches. Measure with a horizontal skinfold.

6. Suprailiac. This site is located halfway between the navel and the top of the hipbone. Measure using a horizontal fold.

7. Abdominals. Measure a vertical fold slightly more than one inch to the side of and one inch below the navel.

8. Thigh. Measure a vertical fold in the center of the thigh, midway between the kneecap and the hip.

9. Medial calf. For this measurement, sit with your right knee flexed at a 90-degree angle and your feet flat on the floor. Using a vertical fold, the measurement is taken on the outer portion of the calf, about midway between the ankle and the knee.

To make your calculations, use the following formula, along with the worksheet in Table 6-2:

1. Add the nine measurements.

2. Divide that total by your bodyweight. This figure gives you the ratio of body fat to bodyweight.

3. Multiply that ratio by .27 to get your percentage of body fat.

4. Multiply your percentage of body fat by your bodyweight to get your pounds of body fat.

5. Subtract the pounds of body fat from your total body weight to calculate the pounds of lean mass.

Body Composition Worksheet — Nine-Point System

Name:_____

Date: _____ Weight: _____

Measurements

Chest _____	Biceps _____
Triceps _____	Subscapular_____
Adominals _____	Thigh _____
Kidney_____	Medial Calf _____
Suprailiac _____	

Calculations

- Total Skinfolds = _____
- Ratio of Body Fat To Bodyweight = _____
  (total skinfolds divided by bodyweight)
- Body Fat Percentage = _____
  (ratio x .27)
- Pounds Of Body Fat = _____
  (body fat percentage x bodyweight)
- Pounds Of Lean Mass = _____
  (bodyweight - pounds of body fat)

Table 6-2

Ideal Body Fat Ranges

"Ideal body fat" is best defined by a range specifying fat content on the body. Here are some ideal ranges to shoot for as you participate in the Lean Bodies Workout.

Well-conditioned men: under 12 percent

Normally active men: 13 to 16 percent

Well-conditioned women: under 18 percent

Normally active women: 19 to 24 percent

"Obesity" usually refers to a body fat percentage that is more than 25 percent for a man and more than 35 percent for a woman.

Goal-Setting On The Lean Bodies Workout

To succeed on the Lean Bodies Workout, you have to be "internally" motivated — driven by goals that are personally important to you.

Suppose your spouse or companion hints that you need to lose weight. So you cut your calories and start an exercise program. While everyone in your family or circle of friends is having "normal" food, you are eating a few leaves of lettuce and a sliver of chicken on your calorie-restrictive diet. While everyone is relaxing or playing at the end of the day, you're sweating it out in the gym. And not liking it one bit.

The reason you are not enjoying your fitness program is because external pressures are motivating you (you are also cutting calories when you should be increasing them). These methods generally don't work, or if they do, it's not for long. So set personal goals — goals you've identified and want to reach. Do it for yourself first; others will be pleased once they see what you've accomplished.

With that in mind, I recommend setting two kinds of goals. The first is a body composition goal. Let's say, for example, that you want to decrease your percentage of body fat and increase your percentage of lean muscle by the end of the eight-week period. In writing your goal, you would state: By [date], my goal is to decrease my body fat percentage to _____ and increase my lean mass percentage by_____.

You don't even have to get that technical. Maybe your body

composition goal is to get down to a smaller dress or pants size. That's exactly what Kathy S. did. Her goal was to fit into a certain set of blue jean shorts. She stepped up the intensity of her weight training program, and concentrated on eating five meals a day instead of three. Before long, Kathy eased into those shorts. Achieving that goal, she says, was "the greatest motivation to continue."

Goal number two is a "performance goal," and you may have several. They should be very specific. Here are some examples: working up to 45 minutes of aerobics a day, entering a 10K race, weight training three times a week, or running a marathon.

Be sure your goals are realistic, too. Sue S. did just that. Her goals were to learn how to work out with free weights and to be able to lift anything in the gym, like the large 45-pound bar. Sue had no trouble reaching her goals. "I can lift that bar without much difficulty. It feels good to be strong enough to lift groceries out of the car without waiting for my husband to come home. Plus, I look firmer and trimmer."

Also, performance goals generally change from week to week, especially since you are striving to work out harder each week. At the start of a week, re-evaluate your goals, whether or not you met them, and then set new performance goals for the week.

Chart Your Progress

Dedicated, successful athletes write down their game plan for nutrition, goals, and training. This is all part of the athletic mind-set — secret #5 for losing body fat.

I want you to write down your game plan, too. You will learn a lot about how your body responds to different nutrition and exercise variables, what works best, how you are progressing in terms of exercise intensity, and how well you are meeting your goals. A game plan committed to paper is a great motivator, too, one that helps you stay on track. Here are several templates you can use to chart your progress. For convenience, they're designed to fit in a regular daytime scheduling book.

GOALS

START DATE:

BODY COMPOSITION GOAL:

BENEFITS OF REACHING THIS GOAL:

STEPS I'M TAKING TO REACH THIS GOAL:

PERFORMANCE GOAL:

WEEK OF:

BENEFITS OF REACHING THIS GOAL:

STEPS I'M TAKING TO REACH THIS GOAL:

PERFORMANCE GOAL:

WEEK OF:

BENEFITS OF REACHING THIS GOAL:

STEPS I'M TAKING TO REACH THIS GOAL:

ATHLETE'S CALENDAR   MONTH: _____

SUNDAY	MONDAY	TUESDAY	WEDNESDAY

BODYWEIGHT:

BODY COMPOSITION:

THURSDAY	FRIDAY	SATURDAY	GOALS

SPECIAL NOTES:

MENU PLAN

DATE:

MEAL:	FOODS:	CALORIES:
BREAKFAST:		
MINI/MOCK MEAL:		
LUNCH:		
MINI/MOCK MEAL:		
DINNER:		

WORKOUT

DATE:

RESTING HEART RATE: **TARGET HEART RATE:**

EXERCISE:	SETS/REPS:	POUNDAGE:

AEROBICS:	TIME/DISTANCE:	TIME OF DAY:

Part II

From Fat To Fit In 8 Weeks

7

CHAPTER SEVEN

The 8-Week Lean Bodies Workout

IN OUR LEAN BODIES CLASSES and through my research, I've found that when it comes to exercise and diet, most people like to be told exactly what to do. Put another way, they like structure. Once you have structure, there are no gray areas or room for guesswork. You know exactly what to do and how to do it. That's how the Lean Bodies Workout is set up.

On the fold-out page that follows is the entire 8-week workout. I suggest that you take the information provided on this sheet and transfer it to your Athlete's Calendar in order to schedule the days and times you'll do your aerobic exercise and your weight training throughout the entire eight weeks. The instructions for exercise performance, guidelines, and routines directly follow the 8-Week Workout in Chapters 8, 9, and 10. Be sure to employ the fat-burning techniques discussed in Chapter 11.

Also on the fold-out sheet you will find exact instructions for increasing your exercise intensity, frequency, and duration each week. As these variables increase, so should your calories. Each week, you will up your calories by 100 if you're a woman; 200 if you are a man. The reason is, you need more energy from food to fuel your higher-intensity exercise. Also, use the Optimal Fueling Formula in Chapter 14 to figure out what your maximum number of daily calories should be for your sex and activity level.

If you haven't already, skip ahead to Chapters 13 and 14 to learn about the Lean Bodies eating program. For a more in-depth discussion of this program, consult the first Lean Bodies book and the Lean Bodies Cookbook. Have your body composition checked, too, so you can track your progress on the Lean Bodies Workout.

Follow this workout exactly as outlined, and within eight weeks' time, you'll be a Lean Body, too. So — off with the body fat, and on with body-shaping muscle!

Week	*Aerobic Intensity	*Weight Training Intensity	*Calories
1	3 sessions, 20 minutes each. Breathe hard enough, yet be able to carry on a conversation.	2 sessions. Use light poundages and concentrate on strict form.	Women: Start with a base diet of 1,500 calories. Men: a base diet of 2,000 calories.
2	3 sessions, 30 minutes each. Breathe hard enough, yet be able to carry on a conversation. (Measure the distance covered; this is your course.)	2 sessions. Choose a poundage you can easily manage for 15 repetitions with good form.	Women: Add 100 calories. Men: Add 200 calories.
3	3 sessions, 30 minutes each. At the end of your sessions, add another 5 minutes at a reduced working pace.	2 sessions. Choose a poundage that lets you get 12 repetitions, but no more, on each exercise set.	Women: Add 100 calories. Men: Add 200 calories.
4	3 sessions, 30 minutes each at a quicker pace, followed by 10 additional minutes at a reduced working pace.	2 sessions. Stick with last week's poundages until you can achieve 15 repetitions with good form.	Women: Add 100 calories. Men: Add 200 calories.
5	3 sessions, 30 minutes each at last week's pace, followed by 15 minutes at a reduced working pace.	2 sessions. Choose heavier poundages that let you get 12 repetitions with good form.	Women: Add 100 calories. Men: Add 200 calories.
6	3 sessions, 30 minutes each, at a quicker pace, followed by 15 minutes at a reduced working pace.	2 sessions. Stick with last week's poundages until you can get 15 repetitions with good form.	Women: Add 100 calories. Men: Add 200 calories.
7	3 sessions, 45 minutes each. Maintain your intensity for 40 of the 45 minutes.	2 sessions. Choose heavier poundages that let you get 12 repetitions, no more.	Women: Add 100 calories. Men: Add 200 calories.
8	3 sessions, 45 minutes each. Maintain your intensity for 40 to 45 minutes.	2 sessions. Stick with last week's weight until you can get 15 repetitions with good form.	Women: Add 100 calories. Men: Add 200 calories.
NOTES	*You may not be able to advance exactly as the 8-Week Workout is set up. Progress at your own rate.	*Follow one of the routines found in Chapter 9. Your goal is to increase your weight training intensity by increasing the poundages you lift. However, you may not be able to increase intensity as the 8-Week Workout calls for. Progress at your own level. If you can't increase poundages, try increasing the number of repetitions you can do.	* Consult Chapter 13 or the first Lean Bodies book to learn how to increase calories from the proper foods. Also, check Optimal Fueling Formula on page X to figure your maximal calorie count.

8

Lean Bodies
Weight Training Exercises

THE BEST WEIGHT TRAINING PROGRAMS employ simple, easy-to-perform exercises. The easier the exercises, the more likely you are to stick with the workout and enjoy yourself while following it. The exercises I've chosen are safe, effective, and designed to produce body-firming, body-strengthening results. They work specific muscles or groups of muscles. In the next chapter, you will see how these exercises are combined to form a "routine," a grouping of exercises.

Equipment

The Lean Bodies weight training exercises employ several different pieces of equipment. They are as follows:

• Barbell: This is a free weight comprised of a long bar with adjustable or fixed plates at each end. On adjustable barbells, the plates are held in place by circular fittings called "collars," which keep the plates from sliding off. For safety, always use collars. Barbells are an excellent type of equipment to have on hand for home weight training.

• Cable Machine: Usually found in gyms and health clubs, cable machines feature pulleys attached to adjustable weight stacks. A variety of grips and handles can be used with cable machines. These machines are often grouped together in multi-station units, some of which are compact enough for home use.

• Dumbbell: This is another type of free weight and is a short bar with adjustable or fixed weights at each end. Collars should always be used with adjustable dumbbells.

• Generic Equipment: This includes exercise benches, slant boards, and chinning bars.

• Plates: These are disc-shaped weights used on barbells, dumbbells, and plate-loading machines.

• Plate-Loading Machine: On this type of equipment, poundage changes are made by loading plates onto a bar on the machine. The leg press is a good example of a plate-loading machine.

• Weight Stack Machine: This refers to weight training equipment that employs a stack of weights that can be adjusted according to the poundage you want to lift. Adjustments are made by inserting a pin into the stack. Leg curl and leg extension machines are examples of weight stack machines.

The Exercises

Each of the exercises below is illustrated by a photograph in this chapter. Be sure to study the photos carefully to get a mind's picture of how the exercise is performed.

Leg Press (Thighs and Buttocks)

1. Load the appropriate poundage on the leg press machine.

2. Position yourself in the machine with your feet resting on the foot platform in front of you. Make sure your knees don't extend past the plane of your feet. Release the safety stops to begin the exercise. Women should not place their feet any narrower than their hips.

3. Slowly lower the platform to about a 90° angle at the knee

joint, and bring your knees toward your chest. Keep your knees in line with your feet.

4. From this position, press the platform back up until your legs are almost straight. Don't lock your knees.

5. Repeat step 3. Continue the exercise for the required number of sets and repetitions.

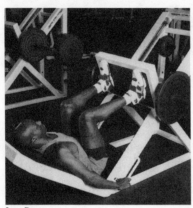 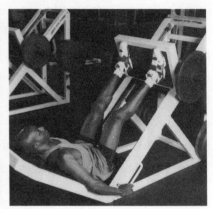

LEG PRESS

Lunge (Thighs and Buttocks)

1. Stand with your feet in a scissor position, as shown in the photograph.

2. Keeping your back straight, lower your body on your front foot until your thigh is parallel to the floor. Your knee should stay over your foot, and your lower leg should not be perpendicular to the floor, as the photograph shows.

3. Push your body back to the starting position, using the strength of your front leg only. Don't lock your knee at the top of the movement.

4. Continue lunging on your front leg for the required number of repetitions. Repeat the exercise on the other leg. To increase the intensity of this exercise, use dumbbells held at your

side or place a light barbell behind your neck across the top of your upper shoulders.

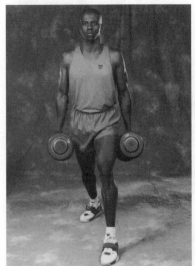 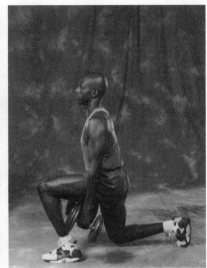

LUNGE

Squats (Thighs and Buttocks)

1. Before performing this exercise, check with your physician if you have lower back or cervical spine problems.

2. This exercise should be performed with the use of a squat rack. A squat rack holds the barbell in place and has catches near the bottom in case you should fail to complete a lift. The barbell should be "racked" or positioned on the rack at shoulder height.

3. Stand facing the bar with your feet about shoulder-width apart. Different foot widths, however, target different portions of the lower body. A wide stance, for example, works the inner thighs and the gluteal muscles (glutes) of the hips; a close stance works the outer thighs.

4. Take a medium overhand grip on the bar. Position yourself underneath the bar so that it's draped across your back shoulders

(the trapezius muscles). Then step back from the rack.

5. Keeping your back as straight as possible throughout the exercise and your eyes focused on a fixed location, bend your knees to a point where the frontal thigh is parallel to the floor. Do not bounce. Your knees and shoulder should not break the plane of your feet. When descending, always sit back.

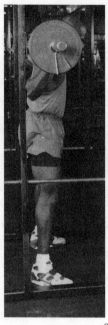
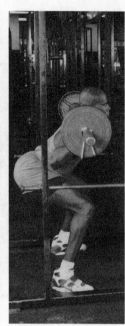

SQUATS

6. Slowly return to the starting position, using the strength of your thighs and hips, not your back. Don't lock your knees at the top.

7. Repeat step 3, and continue the exercise for the required number of sets and repetitions.

Leg Extensions (Frontal Thighs)

1. Select your poundage by placing the pin in the weight stack. (Some leg extension machines are plate-loaded, so you'll have to select the appropriate plate.)

2. Sit in the machine, and hook your ankles under the padded roller.

3. Extend your lower legs up in an arc until your legs are straight. Hold your legs in this contracted position for a few seconds.

4. Slowly lower your legs to the starting position, without letting the weight touch the stack. Continue the exercise for the required number of sets and repetitions.

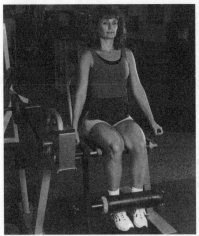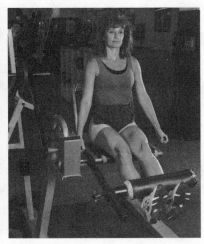

LEG EXTENSION

Note: Many rehabilitation centers are no longer using leg extensions; however, if you have been performing this exercise with good results and no physical problems, continue to use it.

Leg Curl (Hamstrings and Buttocks)

1. Select the appropriate poundage by placing the pin in the weight stack.

2. Lie face down on the machine's bench so that your knees and lower legs overhang it slightly. Your kneecap should not be in contact with the bench. Hook your ankles under the padded roller.

3. Curl your lower legs up toward your buttocks. Keep your hips pressed into the bench during the exercise. Between repetitions, don't let the weights come to rest on the stack.

4. Slowly lower legs to the starting position, and continue the exercise for the required number of sets and repetitions.

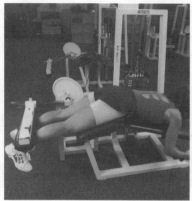 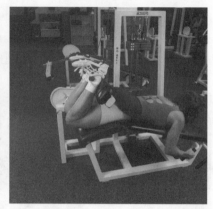

LEG CURL

Bench Press (Chest, Frontal Shoulder, And Triceps)

1. Lie on your back on a flat exercise bench. Have someone hand you the barbell, or lift it off the rack at the head of the bench. Grip width may vary.

2. Begin the exercise with the barbell in a position over your shoulders with your arms straight.

3. From this overhead position, slowly lower the bar to your chest. Don't bounce the bar at the bottom of the movement.

4. Press the barbell back up to the overhead position, stopping just before locking out your elbows. Press your sternum (breastplate) up while squeezing your shoulders down toward the bench.

5. Repeat step 3, and continue the exercise for the required number of sets and repetitions. For a greater range of motion and less stress on the shoulder joint, this exercise can be performed with dumbbells. Any bench press-type exercise can also be performed on an incline or decline bench.

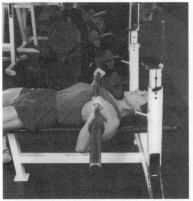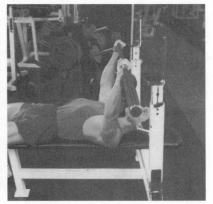

BENCH PRESS

Chest Press Machine (Chest, Frontal Shoulder, And Triceps)

1. Depending on the design of the machine, you'll lie on your back or sit vertically to perform this exercise. To begin, select the appropriate weight on the weight stack.

2. Place your hands on the bar, using a grip that's slightly wider than shoulder-width. Press upward (or outward if you're sitting vertically in the machine) to an overhead position, stopping just short of locking out your elbows.

3. Slowly lower to the starting position, and repeat the exercise for the required number of sets and repetitions.

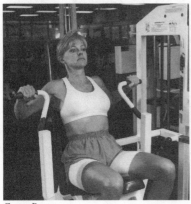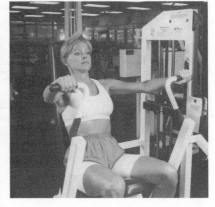

CHEST PRESS

Note: These machines don't fit all body types and therefore may place too much stress on the shoulder joint. This exercise is less effective compared to free weights. Free weights offer better muscle stimulation, particularly on the lowering (or eccentric) portion of the exercise, than machines do.

Dumbbell Fly (Chest, Frontal Shoulder)

1. Hold a dumbbell in each hand, and lie back on a flat exercise bench. Begin with the dumbbells over your shoulder, and your arms slightly bent. The palms of your hands should be facing each other.

2. Lower your arms to your sides in a semicircular motion as far as is comfortable. Strive to get a good stretch in your chest in the lowered position. Keep your elbows pointed out to the side.

3. Still keeping your arms in a semicircular motion, slowly return the dumbbells to the starting position, about six inches apart. Flex your chest muscles in this position. Continue the exercise for the required number of repetitions. The dumbbell fly exercise can also be performed on an incline or decline bench.

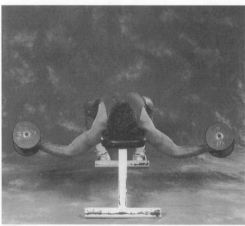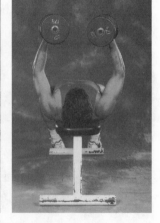

DUMBBELL FLY

Machine Fly (Chest, Frontal Shoulder)

1. Select the appropriate weight by inserting the pin in the weight stack.

2. Sit with your back to the machine's grip handles or pad, and place the bend of your arms on the pads. Never place your forearms on the pads, as this placement can injure the shoulder. Keep your arms in the same position as you would in a dumbbell fly.

3. In a semicircular motion, bring the pads together in front of your body so that they touch. Squeeze your chest muscles in this contracted position.

4. Slowly return to the starting position, and continue the exercise for the required number of repetitions.

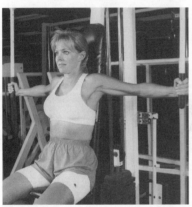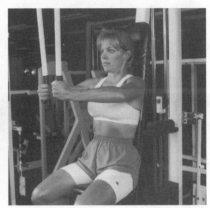

MACHINE FLY

Chins (Upper And Mid-Back, Biceps, And Forearms)

1. Before performing this exercise, warm up on a pulldown machine using a light weight.

2. Take an overhand grip that is slightly wider than your shoulders or an underhand grip that is narrower than shoulder-width. Keeping your knees bent, pull yourself up to the bar. Try to touch your upper chest to the bar, if possible.

3. Lower yourself and return to a hanging position. Throughout the exercise, try to keep your back slightly arched (hyperextended). Try to keep from swinging your body. Continue the exercise for the required number of repetitions.

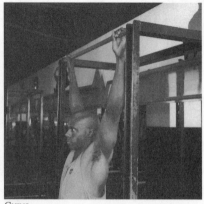

CHINS

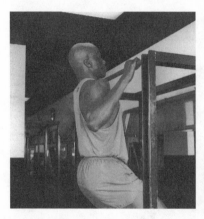

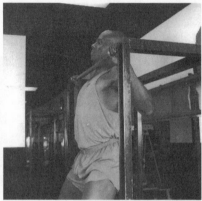

Front Pulldown (Upper And Mid-Back, Biceps, And Forearms)

1. Select the appropriate poundage by inserting the pin in the weight stack located on the pulley cable machine.

2. Sit or kneel facing the machine, and take an overhand grip on the pulley bar that's slightly wider than shoulder-width or an underhand grip that's shorter than shoulder-width. Instead of a pulley bar, you may use a device called a "parallel grip handle."

3. Lean back slightly, and pull the bar straight down, touching

your chest just below your collarbone. Keep your chest up; don't let it cave in.

4. Slowly return the bar to the starting position.

5. Continue the exercise for the required number of sets and repetitions.

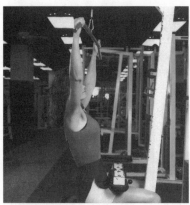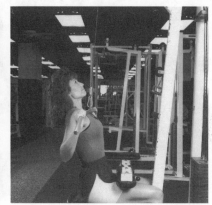

FRONT PULLDOWN

Seated Row (Upper, Mid, And Lower Back, Biceps, And Forearms)

1. Select the appropriate poundage by inserting the pin in the weight stack located on the pulley cable machine.

2. Sit on the bench facing the cable machine and lean forward while keeping your back straight. Grasp the pulley handles.

3. As you slowly sit up, pull the handles in toward your mid-section. Straighten up, and press your shoulders backward, arching your back slightly. Never jerk the weight during the exercise.

4. Lean forward again, returning to the starting position. Try to get a good stretch in this position.

5. Continue the exercise for the required number of sets and repetitions.

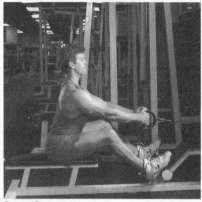
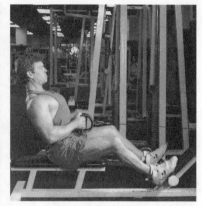

SEATED ROW

Dumbbell Row (Upper And Mid-Back, Biceps, And Forearms)

1. For support, place your knee on a flat bench, with your arm holding onto the bench. Place your other leg slightly behind you. Keep your knee unlocked, and lean on the bench for support. *(Note: Always start with your weaker arm.)*

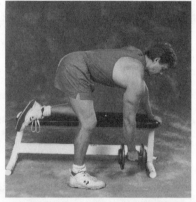

2. Begin with your arm straight (extended), holding a dumbbell. Then pull the dumbbell up to the side of your midsection, raising your elbow as far as possible. Keep your back flat throughout the exercise.

3. Lower the dumbbell to the starting position.

4. Continue the exercise for

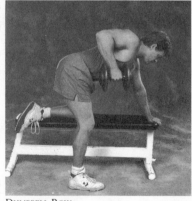

DUMBBELL ROW

the required number of repetitions. Then repeat the exercise with the other arm.

Floor Hyperextensions (Lower Back)

1. Lie face down on the floor with your hands behind you at your sides.

2. Keeping your legs and feet on the floor, slowly lift your head and shoulders off the floor. Then raise your chest off the floor, keeping your shoulders back. Come up as far as is comfortable, then pause.

3. Slowly lower until your chest touches the floor, keeping your shoulders and head off the floor. During the exercise, don't relax your lower back muscles.

4. Continue the exercise for the required number of sets and repetitions.

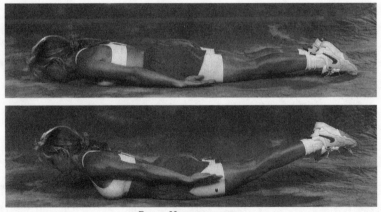

FLOOR HYPEREXTENSIONS

Seated Dumbbell Shoulder Press (Frontal Shoulders)

1. Sit erect on an exercise bench or chair that has back support. With a dumbbell in each hand, begin with the weights at shoulder level, palms facing forward.

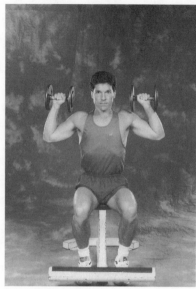
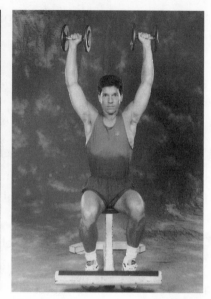

SEATED DUMBBELL SHOULDER PRESS

2. Press the dumbbells up to an overhead position, stopping just before a full lockout of your elbows.

3. Slowly lower to the starting position, and repeat the exercise for the required number of sets and repetitions. This exercise can also be performed with a barbell.

(Note: If you have any lower back or shoulder problems, don't perform this exercise.)

Machine Lateral Raise (Lateral Shoulders)

1. Select the appropriate poundage by inserting the pin in the machine's weight stack. This exercise can also be performed while seated.

2. Place your elbows under the pads.

3. Raise the pads to a position just higher than shoulder level.

4. Slowly lower the pads to the starting position, and continue the exercise for the required number of sets and repetitions.

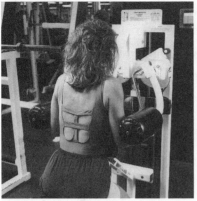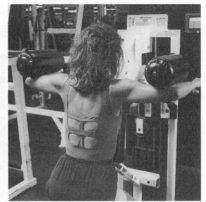

MACHINE LATERAL RAISE

Dumbbell Lateral Raise (Lateral Shoulders)

1. In a standing or seated position, hold a dumbbell in each hand alongside your body, and stand with your feet a comfortable distance apart.

2. Bend your elbows slightly, and raise them up at your sides to a position just slightly higher than shoulder level. Don't let the dumbbells go higher than your elbows.

3. Slowly lower the dumbbells to the starting position, and repeat the exercise for the required number of sets and repetitions.

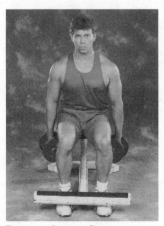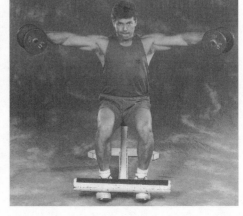

DUMBBELL LATERAL RAISE

Upright Row
(Trapezius, Shoulders, Biceps, And Forearms)

1. Take an overhand grip on the barbell with your hands about 6 to 18 inches apart. Using a "cambered" or E-Z curl bar (a bar that's wavy) is easier on your wrists. Begin with the barbell resting against your upper thighs. Stand with your feet a comfortable distance apart.

2. Slowly raise the barbell straight up to chin-level.

3. Slowly lower the barbell to the starting position, and continue the exercise for the required number of sets and repetitions.

4. This exercise may be performed with dumbbells or with a bar attached to a low pulley on a cable machine.

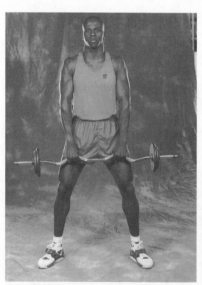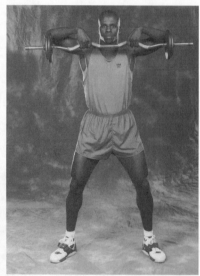

UPRIGHT ROW

Pushdowns (Triceps)

1. Select an appropriate weight, and insert the pin in the weight stack.

2. Stand facing the cable machine, and grasp the high pulley

bar handle with a close, overhand grip and your thumbs on top. Keep your upper arms pressed close to the sides of your body.

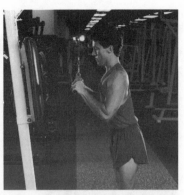

3. Press the bar down until your arms are straight and your elbows locked. Try not to pull the bar into your body. Instead, push straight down so your elbows can lock.

4. Slowly return the bar to the starting position.

5. Continue the exercise for the required number of sets and repetitions. There are a variety of handles you can use on this exercise to reduce stress on your wrists. Experiment with various options to see which you like best.

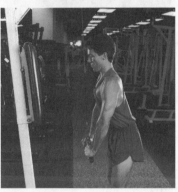

PUSHDOWNS

Overhead Triceps Extension (Triceps)

1. Sit on an exercise bench or chair that has back support. Hold a dumbbell at arm's length overhead.

2. Keeping your upper arms stationary and close to your head, bend your elbow so that your forearms lower behind your head. Your elbows should also remain stationary and pointing toward the ceiling. Make sure the dumbbell doesn't touch your spine.

3. Extend back up to the starting position and lock your elbows at the top. Continue the exercise for the required number of sets and repetitions.

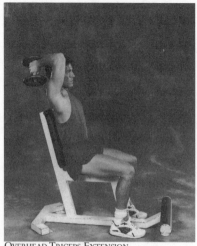

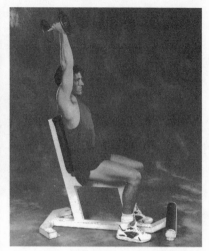

OVERHEAD TRICEPS EXTENSION

Lying Extensions (Triceps)

1. Lie on your back on a flat exercise bench, and have someone hand you a barbell. Take a close, overhand grip on the barbell. Begin the exercise with the barbell over your forehead with your arms straight.

2. Bend your elbows, bringing the bar just behind the top of your head. As you lower the bar keep your elbows pointing forward and your upper arms angled back slightly.

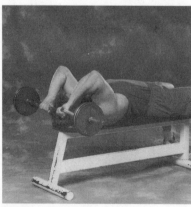

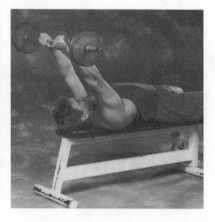

LYING EXTENSIONS

3. Slowly return the barbell to the overhead position.

4. Repeat step 2, and continue the exercise for the required number of sets and repetitions. This exercise can be performed with two dumbbells or a bar attached to a low pulley on a cable machine.

Close-Grip Bench Press (Triceps)

1. Lie on your back on a flat exercise bench. Have someone hand you the barbell, or lift it off the rack at the head of the bench. Using a cambered or E-Z curl bar poses less stress on your wrists.

2. Grip the barbell in the middle with your hands a few inches apart (this grip is more narrow than shoulder-width). Begin the exercise with the barbell in a position over your chest with your arms straight and your elbows locked.

3. From this overhead position, slowly lower the bar to your chest, keeping your elbows close to your sides.

4. Press the barbell back up to the overhead position, and lock your elbows at the top. You should feel the stress on your triceps.

5. Repeat step 3, and continue the exercise for the required number of sets and repetitions.

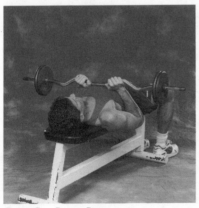 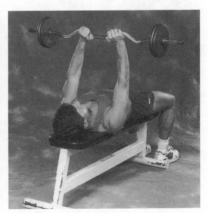

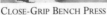
CLOSE-GRIP BENCH PRESS

Chair or Bench Dips (Triceps)

1. With your back to a chair, grasp the sides of the chair or bench and extend your legs out in front of you.

2. Bend your elbows. Then lower your buttocks close to the floor, keeping your elbows close to your sides.

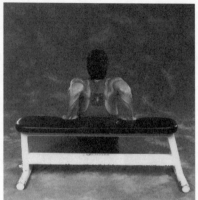

3. After lowering as far as you can, press back up so that your arms are straight and your elbows locked.

4. Repeat step 2, and continue the exercise for the required number of sets and repetitions.

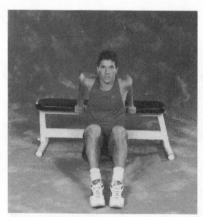
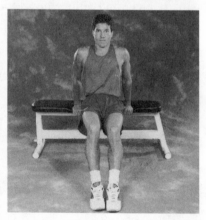

CHAIR OR BENCH DIPS

Barbell Curl (Biceps And Forearms)

1. Take a medium, underhand grip on the barbell. Begin in a standing position with the barbell resting across your upper thighs and your arms straight. Also, keep your back straight.

2. Keeping your upper arms pressed close to your sides, curl the barbell up to chest level.

3. Slowly return the barbell to the starting position.

4. Continue the exercise for the required number of repetitions. You can also perform this exercise with a bar attached to a low pulley on a cable machine.

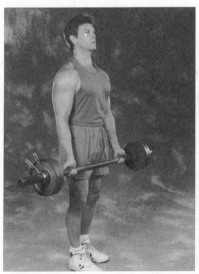 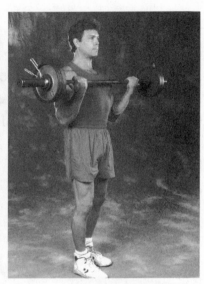

BARBELL CURL

Dumbbell Curl (Biceps and Forearms)

1. For a greater range of motion, use dumbbells in the curl exercise. Begin the exercise with the dumbbells (one in each hand) hanging at your sides with the palms of your hands facing inward. Also, keep your back straight.

2. Curl the dumbbells up to your shoulders. As you do so, make sure to turn your palms so that they face the ceiling.

3. Slowly return the dumbbells to the starting position.

4. Continue the exercise for the 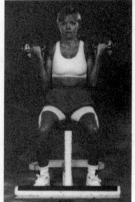 DUMBBELL CURL

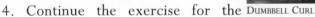

required number of repetitions. You can also perform this exercise with a bar attached to a low pulley on a cable machine.

Preacher Curl (Biceps And Forearms)

1. This exercise requires a special upright apparatus known as a preacher bench that lets you better isolate the biceps muscles of the arm when you're performing curls. The bench should let your arm hang perpendicular to the floor with no angle. Position yourself behind the preacher bench with your arms draped over the front. The top of the bench should fit just under your arms (your armpit area), and your upper arms should be pressed against the bench. Have someone hand you a straight barbell. Begin the exercise with your arms straight.

2. Curl the barbell up toward the top of the bench.

3. Slowly lower the barbell to the starting position.

4. Continue the exercise for the required number of sets and repetitions. This exercise can also be performed with two dumbbells or a bar attached to a low pulley on a cable machine.

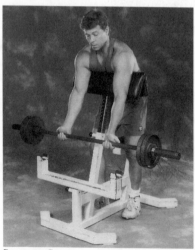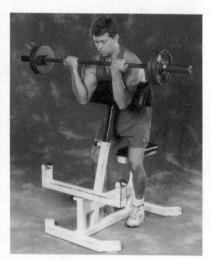

PREACHER CURL

Body Crunch (Abdominals)

1. Lie on your back with your knees bent. Cross your arms over your chest or touch your hands to your temples.

2. Beginning with your shoulders first, lift your upper body off the floor toward your knees. Keep your shoulders off the floor.

3. Slowly return to the starting position. Concentrate on using the strength of your abdominal muscles throughout the range of motion.

4. Continue the exercise for the required number of sets and repetitions.

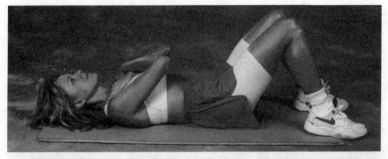
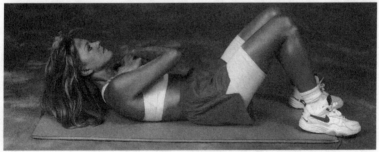

BODY CRUNCH

Machine Crunch (Abdominals)

There are many different kinds of abdominal machines, and each one works somewhat differently. The advantage of these machines is that they easily let you use additional poundages — other than your own bodyweight — to challenge your abdominal muscles to work even harder. Machines with chest pads, however, don't work the abdominals effectively but instead stress a group of muscles called the hip flexors.

I'll give you some basics on how to perform this exercise, but I recommend that you ask a certified trainer or the owner of your workout facility about how to correctly use an abdominal machine.

1. Select the appropriate poundage by inserting the pin in the machine's weight stack.

2. Sit in the machine, and grasp the handles, depending on the design of the machine.

3. Using the strength of your abdominal muscles, shorten your torso by moving your chest toward your hips.

4. Slowly return to the starting position.

5. Continue the exercise for the required number of sets and repetitions.

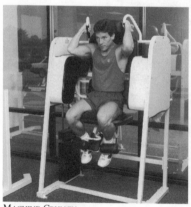 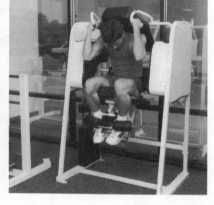

MACHINE CRUNCH

Knee Raise (Abdominals)

1. For this exercise, you'll need a slant board, hanging arm straps, or an apparatus known as a "Roman chair," which features two bars parallel to each other. Depending on which equipment

you use, lie on your back on the slant board, position yourself in the arm straps, or hoist yourself up between the two bars and rest your lower arms on them for support. *(Note: The dip stand form of this exercise is more difficult to perform.)*

2. Bend your knees so that the tops of your thighs are parallel to the floor. Bring your knees up toward your chest. At the top position, your thighs should be slightly higher than parallel to the floor. Try to bring your buttocks up toward your head.

3. Return to the starting position (keep your knees bent — don't straighten them). Repeat the exercise for the required number of sets and repetitions. During the exercise, you should feel the stress on your lower abdominals.

(Note: Avoid this exercise if you feel lower back pain.)

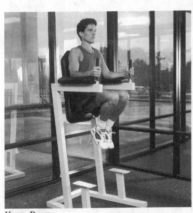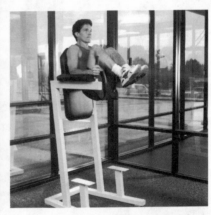

KNEE RAISE

Standing Calf Raise (Calves — Gastrocnemius And Soleus)

1. Select the appropriate poundage by inserting the pin in the weight stack of the machine, or in the case of a plate-loaded machine, by placing a plate on the bar.

2. Step into the machine, and place your shoulders under the pads. The balls of your feet should be on the lower platform with

your heels overhanging it. Keep your knees barely unlocked and your back in the squat position.

3. Slowly raise up on your toes, then lower as far as you can.

4. Continue raising and lowering in this manner for the required number of sets and repetitions.

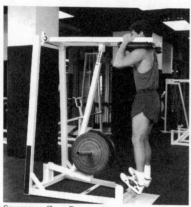
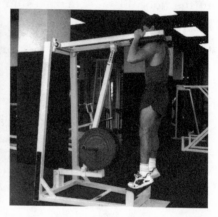

STANDING CALF RAISE

Seated Calf Raise (Calves— Soleus)

1. Most seated calf machines are plate-loaded, so you should begin the exercise by placing the appropriate number of plates on the plate-loading bar.

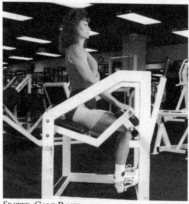
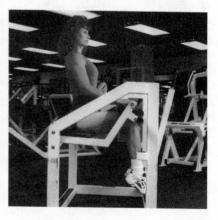

SEATED CALF RAISE

2. Sit in the machine so that the padded bar fits securely across your lower thighs. The balls of your feet should be on the lower platform with your heels overhanging it.

3. Slowly lift your heels, rising up on your toes. Then lower your heels as far as you can.

4. Continue lifting and lowering in this manner for the required number of sets and repetitions.

Toe Raise (Calves)

1. Holding onto a wall or handrail for balance, stand on one leg on a step, and let your heel overhang the step.

2. Slowly raise on your toes, then lower your heels as far as you can.

3. Continue raising and lowering in this manner for the required number of repetitions. Repeat the exercise on the other leg. To increase the intensity of this exercise, hold a dumbbell at your side. You can also perform this exercise on both legs simultaneously.

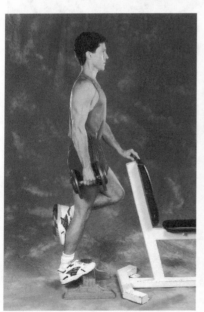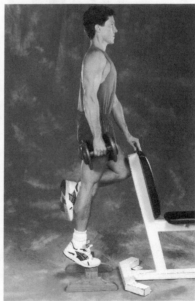

TOE RAISE

Toe Press (Calves)

1. This exercise is performed in a leg press machine. Load the appropriate poundage on the leg press machine.

2. Don't release the safety stops. Position yourself in the machine with the balls of your feet resting on the foot platform in front of you. Your legs should be just short of full knee lockout.

3. With your legs kept straight, press back and forth with your feet, extending your feet and getting a good stretch in both directions.

4. Continue the exercise for the required number of sets and repetitions.

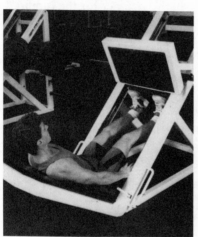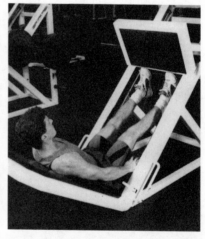

TOE PRESS

9

Lean Bodies
Exercise Routines

THE WEIGHT TRAINING ROUTINES on the Lean Bodies Workout are both time-efficient and easy to follow. There are a total of four routines — two that can be done at home and two that can be done at a gym or health club. Best of all, you use these routines a minimum of twice a week.

They're designed to help you progress slowly, but at a pace that promises results in a few short weeks. If you attempt to do too much too soon, you'll burn yourself out, physically and mentally. Should this happen, you could start dreading your workouts and lose enthusiasm for training. Instead, I want you to look forward to your time in the gym — as something positive and uplifting you're doing for yourself.

Order Of Exercises

Exercise order is an important concept in the Lean Bodies weight training workout. You exercise your large muscle groups first — legs, chest, and back — since they require more energy and effort to train. Small muscle groups like arms and calves are exercised last in the workout. Ordering your workout in this manner maximizes your energy and minimizes fatigue.

The Lean Bodies weight training workout uses the "set system" of training. Exercises for certain muscles are organized into sets. A set is a group of repetitions (the number of times an exercise is performed), punctuated by a half-minute to two-minute rest period.

Warming Up

Generally, there are two ways to warm up prior to starting the Lean Bodies weight training workout. The first is a "general warmup" — light, whole-body exercise that elevates muscle temperature to prepare your body for working out. Walking, using a treadmill, or riding a stationary bicycle for about five minutes are good ways to warm up for weight training.

The second type of warmup is known as a "specific warmup." This involves performing a very light exercise set that warms up a specific muscle or muscle group (as opposed to the entire body). As a warmup for your biceps, for example, you might do an easy 12 to 15 repetitions of arm curls using a light poundage before moving on to your heavier sets.

Many people mistakenly believe that stretching provides a good warmup. But if you stretch a cold muscle, you're setting yourself up for injury. Never stretch a cold muscle. If your toe touching (or anything else) isn't what you'd like in terms of flexibility, then by all means stretch, but do so between exercise sets or after your workout when your muscles are already warm.

Poundages

On most exercises, use the most poundages you can handle for 10 to 15 repetitions each exercise set. This is considered a moderate repetition scheme in weight training. The last two repetitions should feel very heavy. If they don't, then the poundage you are using is too light. Try a poundage that's 5 to 10 pounds heavier. If the poundage feels very heavy the first several repetitions, lighten the weight. Determining the right poundage is often a matter of trial and error. Don't be afraid to experiment, especially as you get stronger.

As noted previously, you begin each exercise with a warmup set using a very light weight with high repetitions. On your next two sets, called "working sets," you'll add more weight (about 5 to 10 pounds heavier) and perform fewer repetitions as the exercise becomes harder.

Never get comfortable with the poundages you're using. Always strive to lift progressively heavier weights. Only by shooting for heavier resistances will you achieve positive changes in your muscles and in your body composition.

Sets And Repetitions

On the Lean Bodies Workout, you will perform two working sets of 12 to 15 repetitions on each exercise. If you can perform more than 15 reps, then increase your poundages. After app. 2 months of training, experiment wieh heavier weights and lower repetitions (10-12 reps). After app. 8 weeks try 6-8 reps for 2-4 weeks then repeat this cycle from the beginning.

Proper Exercise Form

To maximize body mechanics, you must maintain the proper position during your workout. If you need to throw a weight, or contort your body in some way to lift a certain poundage, then the poundage is too heavy for you. That puts you in harm's way of an injury. Stick to poundages that you can lift slowly and smoothly, without sacrificing good form and safety.

Range Of Motion

Range of motion is the full path of an exercise, from extension to contraction and back again. To get the most from every repetition, lift the weight through a complete range of motion.

Also, lower the weight slowly. Research shows that disruption of the most muscular fibrils (the sub-units of muscle fibers) occurs during the lowering phase of an exercise.[2]

Rest And Recovery

Let your muscles rest at least 48 hours following your workout. That's the amount of time required to remove toxins from the muscles and fully replenish muscle glycogen. If you repeatedly train a muscle before its glycogen stores are replenished, you risk damage or loss of muscle tissue. This rest period gives the exercised muscles enough time to recover and rebuild before the next workout.

The Lean Bodies Weight Training Routines

A "routine" is a group of exercises. On the Lean Bodies weight training workout, you can opt to work your entire body (all muscle groups) twice a week or split your routine into three days. Using the split system, you work your upper body two days a week and your lower body one day a week.

*Two-Day Full Body Routine For The Gym

Muscle Groups	Exercise	Sets/Repetitions
Thighs/Buttocks	Leg Press	2 sets of 15 reps
	Leg Extensions	2 sets of 15 reps
	Leg Curl	2 sets of 15 reps
Back	Seated Row	2 sets of 15 reps
	Front Pulldown	2 sets of 15 reps
Chest	Bench Press (barbell or dumbbells)	2 sets of 15 reps
	Flys (machine or dumbbells)	2 sets of 15 reps
Shoulders	Lateral Raise (machine or dumbbells)	2 sets of 15 reps
	Upright Row (cable, barbell, or dumbbells)	2 sets of 15 reps
Triceps	Pushdowns	2 sets of 15 reps
	Lying Extensions (cable, barbell, or dumbbells)	2 sets of 15 reps
Biceps	Standing Barbell or Dumbbell Curl	2 sets of 15 reps
	Preacher Curl (cable, barbell, or dumbbells)	2 sets of 15 reps
Abdominals	Body Crunch (machine or bodyweight)	2 sets of 15 reps
Calves	Calf Raise (standing or seated)	2 sets of 15 reps

Be sure to warm up with 5 minutes of mild aerobics. I also advise performing a very light warmup set before each exercise. This exercise routine shows working sets only.

*Two-Day Full Body Routine For Home Training

Muscle Groups	Exercise	Sets/Repetitions
Thighs/Buttocks	Lunge or	2 sets of 15 reps
	Squats	3 sets of 25 reps
	*Leg curl	2 sets of 15 reps
Back	One-Arm	
	Dumbbell Row	2 sets of 15 reps
	Floor Hyperextensions	2 sets of 15 reps
Chest	Dumbbell Bench Press	2 sets of 15 reps
	Dumbbell Flys	2 sets of 15 reps
Shoulders	Dumbbell Lateral Raise	2 sets of 15 reps
Triceps	Lying Triceps Extensions	2 sets of 15 reps
	Chair Dips	2 sets of 15 reps
Biceps	Standing Barbell or	
	Dumbbell Curl	2 sets of 15 reps
Abdominals	Body Crunch	
	(bodyweight)	2 sets of 25 reps
Calves	Toe Raise (1 leg)	2 sets of 15 reps
	Toe Raise (2 legs)	2 sets of 25 reps

Be sure to warm up with 5 minutes of mild aerobics. I also advise performing a very light warmup set before each exercise. This exercise routine shows working sets only.

*Three-Day Split Routine For Home Training

Muscle Groups	Exercise	Sets/Repetitions
Back	One-Arm	
	Dumbbell Row	2 sets of 15 reps
	Floor Hyperextensions	2 sets of 15 reps
Chest	Dumbbell Bench Press	2 sets of 15 reps
	Dumbbell Flys	2 sets of 15 reps
Shoulders	Dumbbell Lateral Raise	
	or Upright Row	2 sets of 15 reps
Triceps	Lying Triceps Extensions	2 sets of 15 reps
	or Chair Dips	2 sets of 15 reps
Biceps	Standing Barbell or	
	Dumbbell Curl	2 sets of 15 reps

Monday/Friday (Upper Body)

Be sure to warm up with 5 minutes of mild aerobics. I also advise performing a very light warmup set before each exercise. This exercise routine shows working sets only.

*Three-Day Split Routine For Home Training

Muscle Groups	Exercise	Sets/Repetitions
Thighs/Buttocks	Lunge	3 sets of 15 reps
	or Squats using	
	bodyweight only	3 sets of 25 reps
Calves	Toe Raise (1 leg)	2 sets of 15 reps
	Toe Raise (2 legs)	2 sets of 25 reps
*Abdominals	Body Crunch	2 sets of 25 reps

Wednesday (Lower Body)

Do abdominals on one additional day during the week. Be sure to warm up with 5 minutes of mild aerobics. I also advise performing a very light warmup set before each exercise. This exercise routine shows working sets only.

*Three-Day Split Routine For The Gym
Monday/Friday (Upper Body)

Muscle Groups	Exercise	Sets/Repetitions
Back	Seated Row	2 sets of 15 reps
	Front Pulldowns	2 sets of 15 reps
Chest	Bench Press (barbell or dumbbells)	2 sets of 15 reps
	Flys (machine or dumbbells)	2 sets of 15 reps
Shoulders	Dumbbell Overhead Press	2 sets of 15 reps
	Upright Row	2 sets of 15 reps
Triceps	Pushdowns	2 sets of 15 reps
	Lying Extensions (cable, barbell, or dumbbell)	2 sets of 15 reps
Biceps	Preacher Curl	2 sets of 15 reps
	Dumbbell Curl	2 sets of 15 reps

* Be sure to warm up with 5 minutes of mild aerobics. I also advise performing a very light warmup set before each exercise. This exercise routine shows working sets only.

*Three-Day Split Routine For The Gym
Wednesday (Lower Body)

Muscle Groups	Exercise	Sets/Repetitions
Thighs/Buttocks	Leg Press or Squat	2 sets of 15 reps
	Leg Extension	1 set of 15 reps
	Leg Curl	2 sets of 15 reps
Calves	Calf Raise (standing or seated)	2 sets of 15 reps
*Abdominals	Body Crunch (machine or bodyweight)	2 sets of 25 reps

* *Do abdominals on one additional day during the week. Be sure to warm up with 5 minutes of mild aerobics. I also advise performing a very light warmup set before each exercise. This exercise routine shows working sets only.*

10

Your Best Aerobic Bets

ON THE LEAN BODIES WORKOUT, you have many exercise choices when it comes to aerobics. Some of the most popular and effective are:

• Walking
• Jogging
• Running
• Cycling
• Aerobic dance

When selecting an aerobic exercise, make sure it's something you enjoy and are willing to stick with. Whatever you choose, it should be challenging enough to produce plenty of fitness benefits, like fat-burning and cardiovascular improvements. And, you must commit to gradually increasing the intensity of your aerobic effort.

Walking

For anyone just beginning an aerobic exercise program, I recommend walking. Walking has been called the "ideal" exercise — and for good reason. It improves aerobic fitness, burns fat, helps prevent osteoporosis, and cuts the risk of developing coronary heart disease. In fact, research shows that walking nine miles a week throughout your life significantly reduces your chances of developing heart disease.[1] What's more, walking is safe, convenient, and easy to do.

TOTAL FITNESS 131 CLIFF SHEATS LEAN BODIES

To maximize the benefits, a walking program, like any other exercise, must be intense. There are a number of ways to boost the intensity of walking.

• Speed. If you walk at a very fast pace averaging 5 mph, you burn about the same number of calories as jogging.[2] But unless you're a conditioned race walker (an athlete trained in a special mode of fast walking), that speed can be uncomfortable. A more manageable pace is around 3.5 to 4 mph. A 4 mph pace is generally fast enough to elevate your heart rate and keep blood circulating vigorously through your body.

• Distance. You might want to increase your intensity through distance, too. Researchers have looked into the energy costs of walking versus running and found that to burn the same number of calories as running, you need to walk farther.

According to one study, walking expends about 1.15 calories per kg of bodyweight per mile, while running burns 1.7 calories per kg of bodyweight a mile. For example, if you weigh 70 kg (154 pounds), you'll use roughly 80 calories in walking a mile (70 x 1.15) and 120 calories in running the same distance (70 x 1.7). So to burn 120 calories — the same amount as running — you'd have to walk an extra 1/2 mile.[3]

• Frequency. Finally, another way to increase your intensity is by increasing your frequency — the number of times you walk each week.

Guidelines For Walking

1. In hot weather, wear comfortable clothing that fits loosely and allows for good air flow to your skin. In cold weather, dress in layers.

2. Wear well-fitted running shoes to cushion the impact of walking.

3. Warm up with slow walking for three to five minutes.

4. Walk in a safe, well-lit area where these is a smooth surface. Tracks — indoor or outdoor — are ideal. So are indoor malls.

5. Stand erect, with good posture as you walk.

6. When walking, take normal strides but pump your arms in a swinging motion. This pumping action increases the aerobic benefits of walking.

7. Your heel should strike the ground first, then roll onto the ball of your foot.

8. About 10 minutes into your walk, check your pulse.

9. Walk at a brisk pace, so that you are breathing hard but can still carry on a conversation.

10. Try to increase your distance each week. A good rule of thumb, especially for novices, is to start the first week with 20-minute walks. Increase that time by 5 minutes a week until you reach 45 minutes or more.

11. Gradually try to pick up your pace so that you are covering the same distances in less time. For example, shoot for walking 3 miles in 45 minutes (that's about 4 mph), or increase your distance to 4 miles, covered in 70 minutes or less (3.5 mph).

12. Keep records of your progress. Lean Body Jeff R. has an easy way to keep track of his performance. Each morning, he times his morning walk using an athletic watch. After the walk, he records that time on a chalkboard in his garage. Also written on the chalkboard is his best time. His goal is always to beat that time.

13. Take your pulse again at the end of your walk. Your goal is to exercise within your target zone and gradually build your intensity to the higher ranges of that zone. Re-check your pulse after cooling down with slow walking for five to 10 minutes.

14. If you get winded, feel tired, or your pulse rate races, slow down.

Jogging And Running

Walking can be a stepping-stone to higher-intensity activities such as jogging and running. Both are excellent ways to burn fat and achieve cardiovascular fitness, if done consistently. One way to ease into running is with a walk-jog program, a type of workout known as "interval training," in which you intersperse short segments of jogging or running into your walking program. Interval training has some real benefits when it comes to fat-burning and overall fitness. See Chapter 11 for more details.

After awhile, you may be ready to graduate to a full-fledged jogging or running program. The difference between the two has to do with speed. Running is typically any movement over 6 mph.

As with walking, intensity in jogging or running can be increased by picking up your pace, going a greater distance, and increasing the frequency of your runs.

Guidelines For Jogging And Running

1. Wear comfortable but slightly loose-fitting clothing. Your clothing should not restrict your movement.

2. Wear running shoes that are flexible, well-cushioned, and supportive.

3. For safety's sake, never run at night, and always carry some identification. Tell people where you're going.

4. Run on smooth surfaces that minimize impact to the body. Indoor tracks with specially cushioned surfaces, cushioned outdoor tracks, and grassy surfaces are your best bets.

5. Run in an erect (but not stiff) position with your head up.

6. Hold your arms at your sides with elbows bent. Let your elbows swing freely; this helps push your body forward. Stay relaxed, without tensing your limbs.

7. Keep your steps fairly short.

8. Hit the ground with your heel first, rocking your foot forward and then pushing off the ball of your foot.

9. As you jog or run, simply breathe normally.

10. Increase your intensity by picking up your pace or increasing your distance. A word of caution: Running more than thirty miles a week has been associated with increased risk of injury.[4]

11. Check your heart rate during and after your workout.

12. If you get winded, feel tired, or your pulse rate races, slow down.

Treadmills

Treadmills are a popular way to walk or jog. In addition to giving you a great aerobic workout, treadmills work the thighs, calves, and buttocks. The motorized versions let you set the challenge by adjusting the speed of the moving belt, the elevation of its grade, or both. Some models feature digital displays that tell you how many calories you have burned and miles walked.

The non-motorized models are harder to use than their mechanized counterparts. The belt tends to drag, and you end up using energy on pushing rather than walking.

Is there any difference between jogging or running and working out on a treadmill in terms of aerobic capacity? There doesn't seem to be. In one study, eight distance runners ran on both a treadmill and on a track at three different speeds (6.7, 7.8, and 9.7 mph). Researchers could find no differences in aerobic requirements between the two modes of running.[5] In other words: You can get just as much out of treadmill running as you can on the open road or track.

Guidelines For Using A Treadmill

1. Before starting, step on the sides of the machine, not the belt. Once it begins moving, step on the belt carefully.

2. For safety and balance, always hold the handrail.

3. Walk, jog, or run at a pace that keeps up with the speed of the belt.

4. The more conditioned you become, the faster you can go.

5. Use intensity-building features on the machine, such as higher-intensity programs or graded inclines. A word of caution: Walking or jogging on any type of inclined surface has been associated with the increased incidence of shin splints, which are microscopic fractures of the shin bone.

6. To dismount, step on the sides of the machine again and then stop the machine by pushing the appropriate button.

Stairclimbing Machines

Stairclimbing machines involve less impact than running and are greatly respected for a challenging workout.

On most machines, you place your feet on moveable steps, then start stepping up and down. Some models resemble an escalator. You can vary your effort by selecting various intensity levels programmed into the machine.

Guidelines For Using A Stairclimber

1. Be sure to use the warm-up and cool-down features on the machine.

2. Use the handrails for balance only. Letting the weight of your upper body rest on handrails subtracts a lot of fat-burning power from your workout. Slow your pace if you find yourself depending too much on the rails.

3. Place as much of your feet as possible on the steps.

4. Become familiar with the intensity options offered by these machines. Then set up and pursue a program to gradually increase your intensity.

Bicycling

Bicycling is an excellent aerobic activity. It makes your heart stronger and more efficient, burns fat, and strengthens your thighs, calves, and buttocks. Plus, it's gentle on your joints. When you bike at around 20 miles an hour or more on a straight course, you start burning the same amount of calories as you would running 5-minute miles. A drawback of bicycling is the skill level required. You need good balance; finesse in negotiating things in the road, like traffic, holes, and obstructions; and an ability to work the bicycle's gears and brakes properly to accommodate terrain and weather conditions. Even so, bicycling is a top-notch conditioner that can be a lot of fun.

Guidelines For Biking

1. Never take your eyes off the road. Learn to shift gears without looking at them, for example.

2. Learn to use all the components of the bike properly.

3. Learn how to negotiate in traffic — or restrict your biking to less traveled roads.

4. Take your heart rate during and after your ride.

5. Don't wear headphones.

6. Always wear a bicycle helmet.

Stationary Cycling

If you're not enamored with outdoor biking, stationary

cycling may be more your style. Like many types of motorized equipment, these let you select from a variety of programs, each geared to a different level of intensity. Stationary cycling is also an excellent thigh-toner.

Guidelines For Stationary Cycling

1. Adjust the seat height so that your knees are only slightly bent at the lowest point of the revolution.

2. Start with just 15 minutes several times a week. Gradually build up to 45 minutes or more.

3. Experiment with the various program levels on some bikes in order to adjust your intensity level upward.

4. Try to increase the frequency with which you perform your stationary cycling workout.

5. To adequately elevate your heart rate, pedal faster than 60 revolutions a minute or adjust the bike for greater resistance.

Aerobic Dance

More than 23 million people participate in aerobic dance classes each year, making this activity by far the most popular form of aerobic exercise. Aerobic dance is a great fat-burner, it gives an excellent cardiovascular workout, and it works lower body muscles — not to mention that aerobic dance is also fun.

The safest form of aerobic dance is the low-impact variety, in which at least one foot remains on the floor during the aerobic part of the session. Unlike regular aerobic dance, there are no jumps; instead, the exercise uses large upper body movements and relies on kicks, high steps, lunges, and other wide range-of-motion moves. These actions reduce stress on joints, making low-impact aerobics a safer alternative for most people than regular aerobic dance. In many low-impact aerobics classes, hand or ankle weights are added to the exercises to make them more demanding. Stepping up and down on small benches as part of the dance routine is popular, too — and intense.

As with any aerobic activity, be sure to regularly monitor your heart rate while in class to make sure that you are exercising at an appropriate level of intensity. If not, you may want to "graduate" to a higher-intensity class.

Before joining an aerobics class, make sure that the instructors have been certified by a reputable organization and are trained in CPR.

A convenient alternative to attending aerobic dance classes is using exercise videos. They are handy if you don't have a lot of time to spend going from home to class and back again. They are also a good idea if you are self-conscious about going to a health club.

There are drawbacks, however. These include lack of instructor feedback on form and technique, potential injury from working out alone, and lack of the camaraderie you get from an exercise class.

The Cool-Down

For about five minutes following any aerobic exercise, slow your pace by restful walking, light jogging, slow biking, or other mild aerobic activity. This period is called the "cool-down" and should finish off your aerobic workout.

The purpose of the cool-down is to gradually return your heart rate to normal. The best way to do this is by light activity. When you are still in motion, blood lactic acid levels tend to decrease more rapidly, too, accelerating recovery.

Coming Attractions

In the next chapter, you'll learn more about secret #3 — making exercise even more of a fat-burner. It's full of "mini-secrets" about fat-burning. So don't skip this chapter, thinking "you've heard it all before." I guarantee you haven't!

11

10 Ways To Become A Better Fat-Burner

LIKE A LOT OF PEOPLE, Wendy W. had always exercised, but without any dramatic results. That all changed after she came to Lean Bodies. Wendy started the eating program, cutting out processed breads, sugar, and some sweeter fruits and increasing her calories. With leaner eating habits, she was ready to try the Lean Bodies Workout.

"First, I began to do weight training, which I had never done before. Second, I started running in the morning before breakfast — and doing it consistently. The pre-breakfast aerobics recommended on the Lean Bodies Workout really made a difference in my fat loss.

"Today, the intensity of my workouts is about twice as high as before because of my energy levels. I run for 45 minutes in the morning, then another 20 minutes of aerobics after my weight training workout, as Cliff recommends. On the days I don't weight train, I do another hour of aerobics in the afternoon. And, I'm able to run faster."

The results of all this high-intensity effort? Wendy has lost a total of 33 inches and has dropped about six percent of body fat. "Now, because of the Lean Bodies Workout, fat is coming off in all the right places," she says.

Wendy is an example of what I call a "fat-burner." She became one by incorporating a few bona fide fat-busters into her workout.

They worked for Wendy, and they'll work for you. Here's where I let secret #3 out of the bag — how to use proven fat-burning exercise techniques to help you become a better fat-burner too.

1. Turn Up Your Metabolism.

One of the most important ways to become a better fat-burner is to develop your lean mass — your muscle — through regular weight training. Here's a point so important that it bears repeating: Muscle is metabolism. The more you have on your body, the more efficiently you burn calories, even at rest. Imagine this: If you put on just five pounds of muscle, you will burn between 50,000 and 90,000 more calories in one year! Lack of muscle, on the other hand, makes it easy for you to pack on fat pounds.

It doesn't take much time each week to develop muscle, either. On the Lean Bodies Workout, you must exercise with weights at least two times a week. That's just enough time to get the muscular firmness you need to become a better fat-burner.

2. Activate More Muscle.

Activating muscle means to stimulate muscle fibers by overloading them with new demands. The more muscle you can activate during your weight training workout, the faster you'll develop this all-important, fat-burning tissue.

One way to activate more muscle is by approaching "muscular failure." Muscular failure is the point at which you can no longer lift any more weight through a full range of motion. Suppose you are performing a set of dumbbell curls for your biceps. You do the first 10 repetitions with good form, though the effort feels harder as you push through to your goal of 12 repetitions. Finally, you struggle to get the 11th and 12th repetitions. At this point, you have barely enough strength left to lift the weight, but you complete the reps anyway. There's no way you can accomplish a 13th rep. You've reached muscular failure.

Why is this important? At Lean Bodies, we have observed that the last few hard-effort repetitions are "growth stimulators" for the working muscles. In other words, these reps activate more muscle fibers than any of the previous repetitions. Again, the more muscle fibers that are stimulated, the more growth that occurs. And, strong, developed muscle is where the fat-burning action is.

3. Decrease Your Rest Periods.

You can make your weight training workout more aerobic, thus boosting its fat-burning potential, by reducing the time you rest between exercise sets. Most people rest a minute or longer between sets. Try to cut that time down to 30 or 45 seconds. A shorter rest period builds your cardiovascular power and burns more calories.

4. Do Your Aerobics After Weight Training.

As you lift weights, your body is using glycogen from your muscles for fuel. If your weight training session is long — say, 30 to 45 minutes or longer — you can deplete a lot of your glycogen stores by the time the workout is over. Immediately after weight training, you start the aerobic portion of your workout — but with a glycogen-needy body. Theoretically, your body will then be forced to draw on fatty acids sooner for energy during the aerobics. You'll burn more fat, and get leaner as a result.

Even though this response is largely theoretical, people in our Lean Bodies classes who use post-weight training aerobics have experienced great fat-burning results.

There's another advantage, too: Doing aerobics after your

weight training workout spares your strength so that you can lift weights with the intensity you need to develop lean mass. Reversing the order will only sap your strength and compromise your weight training workout.

5. Try Pre-Breakfast Aerobics.

Sleeping through the night is like an all-night fast. When you wake up in the morning, your body is low on glycogen. But what better time to get moving! Rise and shine with 30 minutes of aerobics — before breakfast. With less glycogen, your body has to get fuel from somewhere, so it theoretically starts mobilizing fatty acids from fat stores. More body fat is burned as a result, and you are fast on your way to a leaner physique. We've seen this happen among Lean Bodies clients who regularly perform pre-breakfast aerobics.

There's more: Exercising aerobically first thing in the morning ensures that your metabolism stays cranked up for the rest of the day. Your meals that day are metabolized for energy more efficiently. Plus, the carbohydrates you eat head straight to the glycogen-needy muscles and are less likely to be converted to body fat.

(Note: If you are a cardiac patient, consult your cardiologist on the suitable time of day for performing aerobics.)

6. Try Post-Dinner Aerobics.

Wait for a comfortable time after dinner, then go for a 30-minute run, brisk walk, or other aerobic activity. But afterward, don't eat any carbs. Get a good night's sleep. The next morning, your body will really be glycogen-needy, thanks to the previous night's exercise. After waking up, do another 30 minutes of aerobics — before breakfast. Your body has no choice but to burn extra fat for fuel.

7. Burn More Total Fat Calories With Higher-Intensity Exercise.

A major exercise myth is that lower-intensity workouts, like fast walking, help you knock off fat faster than higher-intensity exercise like running, because the former burns a greater percentage of fat calories for fuel. However, burning a greater percentage of fat calories during exercise doesn't necessarily mean more total body fat loss. With higher-intensity exercise, large withdrawals are made from both fat and carbohydrate stores. When you double your intensity, you practically double the rate at which you burn calories — calories from both fat and carbohydrates. More total body fat is burned as a result.

Case in point: Researchers at the University of Texas discovered that when athletes worked out at only 50 percent of their maximum heart rate, fat supplied 90 percent of the calories burned. When the athletes picked up their pace to 75 percent of their maximum heart rate, fat yielded just 60 percent of calories.

However, the faster, more intense pace actually burned more total fat calories. You see, the 50 percent workout burned only 7 calories a minute, whereas the 75 percent workout burned 14 calories per minute. Here's the arithmetic: The more intense workout expended 8.4 fat calories a minute (60 percent x 14), compared to just 6.3 calories (90 percent x 7).[1]

I don't mean to imply that you must stay in the 70 to 85 percent range for optimum fat-burning! Observing some track athletes, their heart ratios are above the 85 percent level. They are very lean. In my opinion, stepping up your intensity definitely gives you a tremendous fat-burning advantage if you are physically fit enough to push farther on certain days.

8. Gradually Increase The Duration Of Your Exercise Sessions.

If your current level of conditioning doesn't allow you to push for higher intensities just yet, you can still lose fat fast if you gradually increase your duration. One way to do this is by distance traveled. The more distance you go, the more calories you'll burn. Jogging, for example, burns about 100 calories a mile. So if you jogged 2 miles, you'd double your calorie-burning. Increasing distance also increases exercise time. The longer you work out aerobically — 45 minutes or longer — the more fat you'll burn.

9. Increase The Frequency Of Your Exercise Sessions.

Another way to burn more fat is to increase the frequency of your workouts. For example, instead of exercising aerobically three times a week, try doing it five times a week. That way, you increase your total weekly calorie expenditure. For example, let's say you jog three times a week for an hour each time. That's an energy output of about 1,500 calories a week. If you jog two more times a week, you'll burn an additional 1,000 calories, and many of those calories will be fat calories, especially if you're working out at higher intensities. Which brings up this reminder: While increasing either your duration or frequency, always work on upping your intensity as high as you can safely sustain it.

10. Incorporate Interval Training Into Your Aerobic Workout.

Have you ever noticed how lean and defined certain track athletes look? One reason is "interval training," which means alternately speeding up and slowing down during aerobic exercise. During competition and training, track athletes run at three-fourths of their top speed on the straight part of the track, and a slower pace on the curves. Essentially, you can do the same thing — by alternating short bursts of fast running with jogging or walking.

From a fat-burning perspective, the biggest advantage of interval training is that it effectively increases your VO_2 max — with as little as two to four sessions a week.

This has been substantiated by research. In one study, investigators compared the aerobic benefits of interval training with continuous (non-stop) training in two groups of cyclists. The interval group performed 30 seconds of exercise at maximum exercise levels, punctuated by 30 seconds of rest, for 30 minutes a day, three days a week for eight weeks. The other group pedalled continuously (no rest breaks) for the same amount of time and followed the same weekly schedule. The key finding of this study was that interval training produced the greatest increase in VO_2 max.[2]

Boosting your aerobic power in this manner does two things: It creates more fat-burning enzymes and increases the total number and size of mitochondria in muscle cells. This all adds up to greater efficiency in burning nutrients, including fatty acids.

While writing this book, my co-author, Maggie Greenwood-Robinson, decided to incorporate interval training into her workouts. Her goal: to strip off some excess body fat and become more aerobically fit. She started the Lean Bodies Workout at 22 percent body fat and a weight of 133 pounds.

"Because of my writing schedule, the ideal fat-burner for me was to perform aerobics immediately after my weight training workout," she

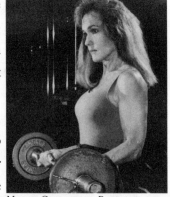

MAGGIE GREENWOOD-ROBINSON

explains. "I knew jogging was a higher intensity form of aerobics, compared to walking, and thus a better fat-burner, but I had always been afraid to try it because of a former knee injury. But the idea of interval training — alternating walking with jogging — appealed to me, so I decided to give it a try. Three to four times a week, I walked-jogged on an indoor track, usually for about 45 minutes each time, always after my weight training session. To my amazement, there was no discomfort to my knee. Interval training was easy to do — and easy to make incremental increases in intensity.

"But the best news of all came when I measured my body fat percentage after six weeks of adding interval training to my workouts. My body fat percentage dropped eight points — to 14 percent — and I've lost six pounds of bodyweight. Now my plans are to pick up my pace and knock a few more percentage points off my body fat measurement."

In addition to fat-burning, there are many other benefits to interval training. For example:

• Interval training can be used to improve endurance in practically every sport — team, individual, and recreational sports.

• Interval training is the best way to develop speed for sports.

• Interval training increases your time to fatigue. In other words, you can exercise longer before you feel the burn of lactic acid buildup.

• Interval training builds strength. Researchers at the University of Wyoming studied cyclists during a six-week interval program, followed by a two-week tapering-off period, and found that the torque strength (the ability to twist or turn forcefully) of their quadriceps muscles (frontal thighs), as well as overall cycling performance, had increased significantly with this mode of training.[3]

• Interval training is fun and motivating, since you are always striving for more speed or distance.

To set up your own personal interval training program, you need to first map out your course. This could be around your block, around an indoor or outdoor track, or down a stretch of unpaved road.

Interval training is divided into the following components, which will help you create your own program:

• Repeats: A specific distance such as one lap or 200 meters or a specific time like one or two minutes that you'll jog, run, or cycle.

• Intervals: The rest period between each repeat. Rest between repeats is performed by walking or jogging, or in the case of cycling, slower-paced pedalling. The purpose of the rest interval is to allow adequate recovery for the higher intensity of the next repeat. During your rest interval, never stop altogether or you'll lose out on the benefits of interval training.

• Repetition: The number of times you perform each repeat.

With interval training, you have the flexibility to vary your workouts for greater intensity and improved fitness. For example, you can lengthen the distance of your repeats, pick up the the pace at which you run them, or shorten the time of your rest intervals. Also, you can increase the number of repetitions you perform during a session of interval training. Following is an example of how to set up a walk/jog interval training program. I suggest that you give it a try as part of your aerobics, then use your imagination to organize your own interval program. Always strive to progressively increase your effort.

*Sample Interval Walk-Jog Program For
The Lean Bodies Workout

Date	Repeats/Intervals	Total Time
Week 1	Walk 1 lap/Jog 1 lap (Repeat several times)	20 - 30 minutes
Week 2	Walk 1 lap/Jog 2 laps (Repeat several times)	20 - 30 minutes
Week 3	Walk 2 laps/Jog 2 laps (Repeat several times)	20 - 30 minutes
Week 4	Walk 2 laps/Jog 3 laps (Repeat several times)	30 - 45 minutes
Week 5	Walk 2 laps/Jog 4 laps (Repeat several times)	30 - 45 minutes
Week 6	Jog 2 laps/Run 3 laps (Repeat several times)	30 - 45 minutes
Week 7	Jog 2 laps/Run 4 laps (Repeat several times)	45 - 60 minutes
Week 8	Jog 3 laps/Run 4 laps (Repeat several times)	45 - 60 minutes

This program should not be followed by beginners, only by more experienced, conditioned exercisers. Also, you may adjust this sample program to fit your level of fitness.

Guidelines:

1. Warm up prior to the intervals by walking for 5 minutes. At the end of your last interval, cool down by walking for another 5 minutes.

2. Try to perform interval training at least three times a week.

3. If a particular week's interval is too taxing, stick to the previous week's interval. Progress at your own rate.

4. Work on increasing your speed and intensity. Try to work within the upper range of your exercising heart rate.

5. Instead of organizing the intervals around laps, you can also set them up according to minutes. For example, walk 2 minutes; jog 3 minutes, gradually increasing the minutes you jog or run each week.

12

Advanced Lean Bodies Weight Training

LONG AFTER THE INITIAL EIGHT WEEKS of following the Lean Bodies Workout and as you become
more experienced in weight training, you may be ready
to experiment with some advanced techniques. There
are a couple of reasons for doing so. First, advanced
training will boost your intensity, further challenging
your muscles to respond. Making a change in your training routine actually shocks muscles into new growth.
Even muscles get bored with the same old stuff! Second,
advanced training keeps your workouts interesting.
There are such a variety of methods to employ that you can't possibly get out of the habit. Advanced techniques are easy to learn
and easy to do. Try incorporating them into your workout program, and you'll be amazed at their body-firming power.

Split Routines

A "split routine" is a short, meaningful training session in
which you exercise only one or more muscle groups at a time.
You've already been introduced to one version of the split routine, in which you exercise your lower body once a week and your
upper body twice a week for a total of three weekly workouts.

To fully understand how a split routine works, picture your
body sectioned off into its major muscle groups — thighs, chest,
back, and so forth. In each workout, you train just one, two, or

three muscle groups at a time. The rationale behind split routines has to do with intensity and recuperation, the process of letting muscles and connective tissue rest and repair before exercising them again.

With split routines, you get the intensity that comes from working just a few muscle groups at a time — and working them harder. The harder you train them, the more they will develop, provided you recuperate adequately between workouts.

Split routines generally allow adequate recuperation. Remember, the time your muscles need for recuperation is at least 48 hours. But connective tissue (joints, tendons, and ligaments) can take even longer. All this means is that you should not train the same body part within that time frame. You can, however, train two or three days in a row if you work different muscle groups on different days. That way, muscles and connective tissue have plenty of time to rest and repair.

There are numerous arrangements of split routines that can be used in weight training. Let's take a closer look at some of the most common ones.

The Four-Day Split

One of the simplest is the four-day split routine, which involves working out four times a week, training each body part twice each week. In the following four-day split, you train your lower body on Monday and your upper body on Tuesday. Skip a day and repeat the sequence on Thursday and Friday. For example:

Four-Day Split Option #1

Monday & Thursday	Tuesday & Friday
Thighs	Chest
Calves	Back
Abdominals	Shoulders
	Arms

Another approach is to work your chest, shoulders, triceps, and hamstrings one day; and your frontal thighs, back, and biceps the next. Skip a day and then repeat the pattern. For example:

Four-Day Split Option #2

Monday & Thursday	Tuesday & Friday
Shoulders	Frontal Thighs
Chest	Back
Triceps	Biceps
Hamstrings	

You can also work your abdominals on separate days, such as Wednesday and Saturday.

Three Days On/One Day Off Split

For even greater intensity and frequency, you might work up to a three days on/one day off routine, if your schedule permits. On this one, you divide your body into thirds, training each muscle group twice a week. The three workouts are punctuated by a day of rest to give your body adequate recuperative time before repeating the cycle. For example:

Three Days On / One Day Off Split

Day 1	Day 2	Day 3	Rest
Chest	Thighs	Shoulders	
Back	Abdominals	Arms	
	Calves		

The Six-Day Split

On a six-day split, each muscle group is trained three times a week. For example:

Six-Day Split

Mon. / Wed. / Fri.	Tue. / Thu. / Sat.	Sun. / Rest
Thighs	Chest	
Calves	Back	
Abdominals	Arms	
	Shoulders	

The above system is more rigorous than the others and may not provide adequate recovery time. At the minimum, muscles need to be trained only once a week to develop properly. So don't think you need to work them three times a week all the time. If you try this advanced workout, do so only for a short period of time.

Every-Other-Day Split

To make sure your muscles are fully recovered before your next routine, try a system called the "every-other-day split." Divide your body in halves as you would with a four-day split. Train the first half one day, followed by a day of rest the next. On the third day, work the second half. Rest again on the fourth day. This method optimizes your energy levels for each subsequent workout.

Time-Saver Three-Day Split

If you don't have time to be in the gym four, five, or six times a week, you can still do a split routine just three times weekly. With this routine, train your whole body one day and then rest a day or two. Your second workout will be devoted to working your upper body; and your third to working your lower body. That way, you train each body part twice a week. For example:

Time-Saver Three-Day Split

Monday*	Wednesday or Thursday	Friday or Saturday
Thighs	Chest	Thighs
Chest	Back	Calves
Back	Shoulders	Abdominals
Shoulders	Arms	
Abdominals		
Arms		
Calves		

Don't train to failure on this day in order to help your body better recover and to conserve strength for the remaining workouts.

Advantages Of Using Split Routines

To the uninitiated, split routines probably seem rigorous and grueling. But there are a number of advantages — both in physical conditioning and in mental attitude toward training.

For starters, a split routine can enhance your efforts to lose body fat. Weight training is an energy-expensive activity that uses up to 500 calories an hour, depending on how hard you work out.

So with extra training days added to your schedule, you expend more calories each week.

By training on a split system, you get a productive return for the time you spend. You can concentrate more fully on each exercise, isolating particular muscles and perfecting your technique, which in turn promotes muscular development.

For some people, split routines may solve exercise motivation problems. You are more likely to stick to an exercise program if you can build it into your daily routine. For a lot of people, being in the gym several times a week is motivationally reinforcing and helps the workout habit become ingrained. It's a good idea to keep your split routine short, however. Otherwise, you could experience the burnout often caused by long workouts. Plus, a short workout leaves you time to do other things afterward, such as aerobics.

Another advantage of split routines is the variety of exercises you perform from workout to workout. Plus, when you get bored with certain exercises, move on to others. That's one of the great things about weight training: There are hundreds of exercises available. This variety of activity is a great way to combat staleness, a real problem among exercisers and one that can lead to exercise dropout.

Putting It All Together

If the split system sounds like something you're ready to try, how do you begin? Consider starting with the four-day split routine to see how it works into your schedule.

Energy level and recuperative ability are important considerations, too. Here you must listen to your body's signals. Persistent fatigue and muscle soreness are signs that you may not be suited to working out five or six times a week.

Finally, your lifestyle is a critical factor. Taking into account your job and family commitments, how many days can you reasonably spend in the gym? The most important point about training is to maintain a balance in your life. That means making time for friends, family, career, and other activities, in addition to fitness.

How To Set Up Your Split Routine

To guide you on structuring your own split routine, here are several split routines, each adaptable to training at home or at a gym. You can follow them exactly as written or modify them for your schedule and the type of equipment available to you. In each routine, the larger muscle groups are worked first, when your energy level is at its peak.

With each set be sure to "pyramid" your weights. As explained previously, this simply means increasing your poundage from set to set. Always perform an initial warmup set with light poundage. Establish your initial poundage by attempting 12 reps using strict form. If you can't make 12 reps with proper form, the weight is probably too heavy. On the other hand, if you can complete 15 without exertion the weight is too light.

Use your workout log, too, in which you record the exercises, the number of sets and reps, and the amount of weight you lift. Charting your achievements is an excellent motivator.

*Four-Day Split

Monday & Thursday		
Thighs/Buttocks	Squat or Leg Press	2 sets of 15 reps
	Leg Extension	2 sets of 15 reps
	Leg Curl	2 sets of 15 reps
Abdominals	Body Crunch	2 sets of 15 reps
	Knee Raise	2 sets of 15 reps
Calves	Standing Calf Raise	3 sets of 15 reps

Tuesday & Friday		
Back	Lat Pulldown	2 sets of 15 reps
	Floor Hyperextension	2 sets of 15 reps
Chest	Dumbbell Bench Press	2 sets of 15 reps
	Dumbbell Flys	2 sets of 15 reps
Shoulders	Dumbbell Shoulder Press	2 sets of 15 reps
	Dumbbell Lateral Raise	2 sets of 15 reps
Triceps	Pushdown	3 sets of 15 reps
Biceps	Barbell Curl	3 sets of 15 reps

* Be sure to warm up with 5 minutes of mild aerobics. I also advise performing a very light warmup set before each exercise. This exercise routine shows working sets only.

*Time-Saver Three-Day Split

Monday		
Thighs/Buttocks	Squat or Leg Press	2 sets of 15 reps
	Leg Curl	2 sets of 15 reps
Back	Front Pulldown	2 sets of 15 reps
	Seated Row	2 sets of 15 reps
Chest	Dumbbell Bench Press	2 sets of 15 reps
	Machine Flys	2 sets of 15 reps
Shoulders	Dumbbell Shoulder Press	2 sets of 15 reps
	Machine Lateral Raise	2 sets of 15 reps
Triceps	Lying Extensions	2 sets of 15 reps
Biceps	Barbell Curl	2 sets of 15 reps
Abdominals	Abdominal Machine	1 set of 25 reps
Calves	Toe Press	2 sets of 15 reps
Wednesday or Thursday		
Back	Front Pulldown	2 sets of 15 reps
	Dumbbell Row	2 sets of 15 reps
Chest	Chest Press Machine	2 sets of 15 reps
	Dumbbell Flys	2 sets of 15 reps
Shoulders	Dumbbell Shoulder Press	2 sets of 15 reps
	Dumbbell Lateral Raise	2 sets of 15 reps
Triceps	Close-Grip Bench Press	2 sets of 15 reps
Biceps	Cable Curls	2 sets of 15 reps

Friday or Saturday		
Thighs/Buttocks	Lunge	2 sets of 15 reps
	Leg Curl	2 sets of 15 reps
Abdominals	Crunch	2 sets of 15 reps
Calves	Seated Calf Raise	3 sets of 15 reps

* Be sure to warm up with 5 minutes of mild aerobics. I also advise performing a very light warmup set before each exercise. This exercise routine shows working sets only.

*Three Days On / One Day Off Split

Day One—Chest and Back	
Exercise	*Sets & Repetitions*
Barbell Bench Press	2 sets of 15 repetitions
Dumbbell Fly	2 sets of 15 repetitions
Front Pulldown	2 sets of 15 repetitions
Seated Row	2 sets of 15 repetitions
Floor Hyperextensions	2 sets of 15 repetitions
Day Two — Legs and Abdominals	
Leg Press or Squat	2 sets of 15 repetitions
Leg Extension or Lunge	2 sets of 15 repetitions
Leg Curl	2 sets of 15 repetitions
Crunch	2 sets of 15 repetitions
Knee-Ups	2 sets of 15 repetitions
Standing Calf Raise	3 sets of 15 repetitions
Day Three—Shoulders and Arms	
Overhead Dumbbell Press	2 sets of 15 repetitions
Dumbbell Lateral Raise	2 sets of 15 repetitions
Pushdown	3 sets of 15 repetitions
Barbell Curl	3 sets of 15 repetitions
Day Four — Rest	
Days Five, Six, & Seven — Repeat Cycle	

* Be sure to warm up with 5 minutes of mild aerobics. I also advise performing a very light warmup set before each exercise. This exercise routine shows working sets only.

Advanced Workout Techniques

Now let's look at a number of training variations that can be used within routines to increase intensity, accentuate fat loss, and keep your workouts from becoming stale.

Forced Reps

When you push yourself so hard that you can't finish the last rep of a set, you've trained to "failure," a concept explained in Chapter 11. A few "forced reps" will help you get past your "failure" plateaus, or sticking points. Have a training partner assist you with forced reps by gently lifting the bar while you continue to push. Forced reps are a good way to progress in your training, but use them only occasionally in your workouts — no more than once a week.

Negatives

In weight training, lowering the bar is referred to as the "negative phase" of the lift, while raising the bar is the "positive phase." Both motions cause the muscle to contract, thus activating muscle fibers. Theoretically, more muscle fibers are disrupted during the negative phase, thus stimulating growth and development. That's why it's so important to control the weight as you lower it.

You can take advantage of this muscular response by periodically performing negative work after you've completed a normal set. For a few repetitions, have your partner first raise the weight for you. You then lower the weight in a slow and controlled manner, resisting its gravitational momentum. Negative training is a good way to build strength in muscles that are weak and lag in development.

Supersets

"Supersets" combine two different exercises, performed without rest in between. Supersets spark muscle growth. Plus, they represent a time-efficient way to exercise and make your workouts more fun to boot. There are several ways to superset exercises:

• Same muscle: On each set, you work the same muscles but use a different exercise. A triset consists of three different exercises and giant sets are made up of four (or even five) different exercises. Some examples:

- Biceps curl/cable biceps curl (regular superset for the arms).

- Barbell bench press/dumbbell bench press on an incline bench/dumbbell fly (triset for the chest).

- Overhead triceps extension/lying extensions/close-grip bench press/ chair or bench dips (giant for the triceps).

• Opposing muscle: Work opposing muscles, such as triceps and biceps, one muscle right after the other with little rest in between. An example would be a set of biceps curls followed immediately by pushdowns for the triceps.

• Pre-exhaustion: Many people get excellent results from a type of superset known as "pre-exhaustion." This technique consists of an "isolation" exercise (an exercise for a specific muscle) immediately followed by a "compound" exercise (one that works a large grouping of muscles). In many compound exercises, smaller, weak-link muscles often give out early, hindering the development of larger muscle groups. Pre-exhaustion solves this problem.

Take the chest, for example. In many chest (pectoral) exercises, the triceps are the weak-link muscles. When you do chest exercises, the triceps are worked hard and the chest muscles just moderately. With pre-exhaustion, first perform a set of dumbbell flys, an exercise in which the triceps are not directly involved, to exhaust the pectoral muscles of the chest. Next, do a set of bench presses. Your triceps are temporarily stronger so you can finish the presses without limitations. Your chest muscles are thus worked to their fullest.

Examples of other pre-exhaustion sets include:

• Lateral raises/overhead shoulder press (shoulders).

• Leg extensions/squats (thighs).

• Push downs/ bench dips (triceps).

Experimenting with supersets and other advanced techniques can take you to new levels of muscular fitness. Just be sure you're eating enough calories every day, and not skimping on important nutrients. That way, you'll continue to make progress and look great.

Part III

Food As Fuel For The Lean Bodies Workout

13

Energize With More Calories

IF YOUR BODY WERE A FERRARI, wouldn't you want to power it with the highest grade, best performing fuel around? Of course you would! To be a lean, high-performance machine, you need the right kind of fuel.

But so many people put in junk instead, and performance and looks both suffer. Take Paula P., for example. She has a highly active lifestyle — she's a dance teacher — but until coming to Lean Bodies, she powered her body with a lot of of fried foods and fast foods. Paula teaches dance classes and is a pupil herself, so she's in class many hours each week. You'd think with that activity level, she would be lean and firm, right? Wrong! Paula needed to lose body fat. She was so uncomfortable with her weight that she would undress in front of her husband with the lights off!

On Lean Bodies, Paula increased her calories to 2,200. "I noticed the biggest difference in my third week when I was in the 2,100 to 2,200 calorie range. My energy level was high, and I wasn't tired by the end of the work day," she says.

The best news of all is that she has lost 14.5 percent of her body fat and 6 pounds altogether. Plus, she has gained 8 pounds of muscle. No longer does she undress in the dark.

Paula plans on continuing Lean Bodies, and she told our staff recently: "Watch out! My lean and mean Ferrari is on the way."

Rethink Your Food Attitude

What does food mean to you?

To some, it means comfort; to others, fun and excitement. We seem to attach all kinds of emotions to food. That attachment gets us into trouble because we eat for the wrong reasons— and often over-indulge in sugary, fatty foods as a result.

I can give you umpteen facts about different types of food, from nutrient content to health effects. But the most important point about food is that it's fuel.

That's right. Food is fuel, pure and simple. Once you start looking at food with this attitude, food will be your servant, not your master. Begin to learn to eat what nourishes and energizes your body, not what comforts or excites it.

Clean-Burning Fuel

The right type of fuel is vital to health, just as the right type of gasoline is for a car. On the Lean Bodies eating program, you eat specific kinds of nutritional fuel: lean proteins, starchy carbohydrates, fibrous vegetables, low-sugar fruits, and essential fatty acids. These are all natural foods, with little, if any, processing and no additives or preservatives either. Pure, unadulterated food.

Why is this such a big deal? Because your body uses natural food so much more efficiently than processed, chemical-laden food. Natural food is put to use in building the body, whereas processed food is more likely to be stored as fat. Put another way, natural food is clean-burning fuel; processed food just gums up the works.

For perspective, consider the foods eaten in Biblical times: plenty of barley and other whole grains, legumes, vegetables and fruits, and seafood — all natural foods. In those days, too, the major mode of transportation was walking, or if you went for a boat ride, you rowed. I consider myself an active person. But if I had lived in Biblical times, I really wouldn't be considered any fitter than the rest of society! All the exercise, all the natural food back then — that lifestyle might be part of the reason why Biblical patriarchs lived such robust and productive lives, well into their eighties and beyond.

Stop Dieting And Increase Calories

Just as important as eating the right foods is the need to gradually increase the calories from those foods. Increasing calories forces your metabolism out of a slack mode into high-gear, so your body can start burning fat more efficiently. The notion of increasing calories is mind-boggling, but it works. At first, you will think you can't possibly eat all that food. It's just too much, you'll say! But soon your metabolism will be so charged up that your system will demand this new, higher level of calories.

To help you change your thoughts about increasing calories, let's look at what happens when you take the traditional approach to losing weight — the cut-calorie method. It's based on the theory that being overweight is caused by overeating. So if you eat less, you'll shed pounds. But wait: Nearly 95 percent of those who go on low-calorie diets regain their weight, plus interest, within five years. Clearly, diets still don't work. In fact, let me give you five reasons why diets make you fat:

(1) *Loss of muscle.* Up to 50 percent of the weight you lose on a diet is muscle, and losing it slows your metabolism.

(2) *The starvation trick.* Cut calories and your body is tricked into thinking it's starving. A special fat storage enzyme called lipoprotein lipase goes to work, signalling your body to stockpile fat once it's fed again.

(3) *Heat energy*. Calorie restriction causes less food energy to be given off as body heat. It's converted to weight instead.

(4) *A slower metabolism*. Food restriction suppresses hormonal action, which in turn makes the metabolism sluggish.

(5) *The rebound effect*. After a diet, fat stores stand first in line to be replaced after dieting.

A Life-Changing Story

Restrictive diets often lead to full-blown eating disorders like anorexia and bulimia. At age 14, Alayne C. started subsisting on 200 to 500 calories a day so she could look "model-thin" — a pattern of starvation that continued on and off for 13 years. "Three years ago, I was watching a television talk show on anorexics, and I realized that was me!"

Alayne began to get migraine headaches in high school. Her mother took her to an eye doctor for treatment, and he warned her that if she continued to lose weight, she could go blind. "That really scared me, so I began gaining weight. However, at the time, I was modeling and was told to lose five pounds. Once again I began losing weight."

Alayne got engaged at age 23. But her joy over the engagement was clouded by her mother's diagnosis of terminal cancer. The emotional turmoil triggered wide swings of yo-yo dieting — up 20 pounds, then back down to a sliverish 109 pounds. To keep from gaining weight, Alayne avoided eating by putting her food in a napkin at meals, then throwing it away.

"Three years later, my mother-in-law told me that if I kept looking the way I did, I would lose my husband," Alayne remembers. "That made me freak out. For the first time, I looked in the mirror and saw that I was too skinny."

Still, Alayne could not pry herself from the clutches of the disorder. She was eating, but her meals consisted of processed bread, butter, and cheese.

After both her children were born, Alayne tried to lose weight again by starving herself. By this time, her metabolism had shut down, and no weight was coming off.

"My husband had heard about Lean Bodies. I called Cliff, and signed up for the program. I learned how to lose body fat by eating more! Cliff taught me to increase my caloric intake and reduce my fat to speed up my metabolism. At first, I was nervous about eating so much food, but I stayed on the program, and for the first time in my life, I'm in control of my health."

Today, Alayne's nourishment gives her the energy to work out aerobically six times a week, along with one hour of weight training three times a week.

"It's amazing what proper nutrition and exercise can do. So many people try to work out as hard as they can and eat as little as possible. Total health requires both exercise and proper nutrition. I'm now 35 years old and have never felt better. I'm no longer afraid to eat, and best of all, I will never have to diet again!"

More Success Stories About Increasing Calories

Does all of this really work? You bet, and before I give you a summary of the eating program, let me share a few more case studies with you.

• Despite being a marathon competitor, Beverly J. couldn't lose body fat — all because she dieted too rigorously. Once she started Lean Bodies, Beverly increased her calories to approximately 2,000 and discovered something amazing. As she puts it: "The more I ate, the more body fat I started losing." She has reduced her body fat from 17.7 percent to 14.9 percent. "The program is now a way of life for me and my family."

• For more than 10 years, Judy P. was caught up in the typical cycle of over-eating followed by panic dieting. It was driving her crazy! "I knew there had to be an easier way to get in control of my diet," she says. (Judy is one of our exercise models in this book, so you can see for yourself how well proper nutrition and exercise work!)

"I started Lean Bodies and knew within the first week it was the answer I was looking for. I had permission to eat again — and I mean really eat. I lost body fat and have gained muscle, but the real bonus is the increase in energy I now have and the great sense of well-being I now feel. It's so easy to be in control!

"The program is for everyone — no matter what your goals!"

• "Following this program has changed my life," says Kathryn M. "It has restored my self-confidence. I look and feel better than I have in many years. The goals I set to get a lean body were easily accomplished on this program. Now I have all the energy needed as a fourth grade teacher and extra energy for after-school activities."

She adds: "This program can help you lose body fat and increase lean muscle, while you enjoy tasty, nutritious foods. The eating habits I've learned will last a lifetime."

I hope these stories are convincing enough to prove how important it is to energize with more calories. In the next chapter, you'll learn how to put meals together to fuel your body the right way.

14

Fueling The Fit Body

AT 5'5", TERI D. WEIGHED 130 POUNDS (not too out of range for her height), but carried 25 percent body fat.

"I signed up for the Lean Bodies classes and did exactly what I was told, as far as starting out at 1,500 calories a day the first week and then increasing my calories by 100 each week after that. I noticed an immediate surge in my energy level and a huge change in my body shape — even before I started the Lean Bodies Workout three weeks later."

Over the course of a year, Teri's body fat percentage steadily fell. Right now, it measures a lean 12.6 percent. Teri was a size 6 or 8 when she started the program, and is now a size 4.

Prior to signing up for Lean Bodies, Teri had not exercised in three years. The energy she experienced from the eating program motivated her to get moving. She now does the Lean Bodies Workout — an hour of aerobics four to five times a week, plus upper and lower body weight training twice a week. What's more, she still has energy left over to do 30 to 40 minutes of toning exercises for her abdominals, thighs, and buttocks four or five times a week.

As Teri learned, gradually increasing your calories from the right foods upgrades your metabolism. You process food so effectively that it's used to build lean tissue. At the same time, your faster metabolism helps burn fat more efficiently.

To give the Lean Bodies Workout 100 percent effort, you need to follow the Lean Bodies eating program. I'll give you the basics here, but I recommend that you obtain a copy of my first book, now in paperback.

Lean Protein

Besides exercise, there's something else that's firming up your body — protein. Protein has gotten a bad rap in nutrition. It's been falsely accused of causing heart disease and other diet-related illnesses. But the real problem is not protein but too much saturated fat, which can contribute to elevated cholesterol levels. Also too little activity is detrimental to cardiovascular health.

On this plan, you eat lean protein, which is low in fat. Lean protein is a good thing for health. Here's why: Every cell in our body relies on protein for life. The lifespan of a red blood cell, for example, is only 18 weeks. Unless it's fed with protein, it won't reproduce.

Our bodies are protein. Dietary protein is used to build bones, organs, nerves, muscles — literally every substance in the body. Each day, you must eat enough protein to exist, regenerate the body, and stay healthy.

Protein And Muscle

As an active person, you should be aware of protein's role in performance. Protein plays a key role in the body's "anabolism/catabolism cycle." Daily activity, including exercise, causes a natural breakdown of muscle tissue, known as catabolism. For muscle tissue to build itself back up and form new tissue (anabolism), the body needs protein for growth and repair.

Here's a simplification of how this cycle works: Tear lean muscle down during exercise. Feed it with protein and other nutrient-rich foods, and it grows back stronger and harder.

Protein And Fat-Burning

Protein is also associated with fat-burning, though most people don't see it that way. In fact, many nutritional experts advise people to eat more carbohydrates so they can lose fat, yet nearly 71 percent of all Americans are overweight. Clearly, something is wrong with this picture!

There's no question that carbohydrates, especially natural, complex carbs, are a nutritional mother lode, supplying energy, fiber, vitamins, and minerals. But too much carb in the diet can hinder fat loss, particularly if you're not very active. A carb overload can trigger a high release of insulin into the bloodstream. Insulin activates fat cell enzymes, facilitating the movement of fat from the bloodstream into fat cells for storage. Additionally, insulin prevents glucagon from entering the bloodstream, and glucagon is responsible for unlocking fat stores. The cumulative result of these interactions is the ready conversion of carbs to body fat.

Therefore, one dietary key to keeping fat storage under wraps is to balance your insulin and glucagon release. You can do this by eating a diet consisting of 20 to 25 percent protein (or more), 60 to 65 percent carbohydrates, and the rest from fat. These are the ratios used on the Lean Bodies eating program. By keeping your carb consumption in this range, you inhibit the release of insulin. This in turn stimulates glucagon, which can then go to work, liberating fat stores.

Once Lean Bodies participants see the difference this eating pattern makes in their ability to lose body fat, they become convinced immediately. As Lean Body and personal trainer Annette P. puts it: "Protein is extremely important, but the need for carbohydrates is severely overrated when trying to stay lean. I'm not saying that carbohydrates are any less important than protein. However, many diets today insist on increasing the intake of carbohydrates. Unless you have an extraordinary metabolism, these diets will not work properly for you."

Protein Choices

Two kinds of protein exist: complete protein and incomplete protein. Complete proteins, found in animal sources of protein, contain all the essential amino acids needed for growth and repair. The body doesn't store essential amino acids, so we have to get them from our food.

Proteins from plant sources are considered "incomplete" because they lack the amino acids essential for building and repairing tissue. Foods such as rice, potatoes, nuts, and grains contain essential amino acids but in lesser quantities than the lean proteins.

Also, animal sources such as the lean proteins are absorbed more efficiently by the body (about 90 to 95 percent) than are proteins from plant sources (73 percent).

Remember, your body is constantly using up amino acids every minute of every day for repair and maintenance, so you must eat essential amino acids every day. In Table 14-1 are the lean animal proteins you may include on the eating program.

LEAN PROTEINS

Amberjack	Non-fat yogurt*
Bass	Ocean catfish
Bluefish	Ocean perch
Chicken, white meat	Pike
Clams	Pollock
Cod	Rainbow trout
Egg whites, cooked	Salmon
Flounder	Sea bass
Game meats	Shad
Grouper	Shrimp
Haddock	Skim milk*
Halibut	Snapper
Trout	Soybeans
Longhorn beef	Sugar-free soy milk
Mackerel	Swordfish
Non-fat cottage cheese*	Tuna
Non-fat tofu*	Turkey, light meat

Table 14-1

These foods are low-fat dairy products. The first eight weeks of the program, limit your intake to 6 to 8 ounces daily.

Carbohydrates

Carbohydrates load your muscles with glycogen, the storage form of carbohydrate. Glycogen is broken down for energy when your body needs it.

Much misunderstanding exists regarding sources of carbohydrates. It's true that donuts, pies, cakes, ice cream, pastries, and snack foods are carbohydrates. These are, however, refined carbohydrates. They give you a quick rush of energy followed by a fast crash into fatigue.

If you want sustained energy, eat complex carbohydrates, not refined carbohydrates. Two types of complex carbohydrates are used in the Lean Bodies eating program: starchy carbohydrates and fibrous vegetables. Starchy carbohydrates are "slow-releasing" foods; that is, they supply a sustained, enduring form of energy that lasts throughout the day, especially when combined with protein in a meal. These foods are also high in quality calories for stimulating the metabolism and keeping energy stores full.

Low in calories, fibrous vegetables supply fiber, water, and most importantly, vitamins and minerals. These nutrients are essential for forming body structures and controlling all the processes required to stay healthy.

Some of the carbohydrates you eat are used for immediate energy, while some will be stored as glycogen in the liver and muscles. After intense exercise, it takes about 48 hours for the body to synthesize glycogen to replenish the muscles. An energy-boosting practice is to re-supply your body with glycogen after exercise by eating starchy carbohydrates with a small amount of protein or drinking a "mock meal" shake as recommended by the program (the mock meal is explained, under "Building Your Meals.")

Remember, about 60 to 65 percent of your daily calories should come from carbohydrates (both starchy carbohydrates and fibrous vegetables). Tables 14-2 and 14-3 list the various carbohydrate choices to incorporate in your daily menus.

STARCHY CARBOHYDRATES

Barley	Cream of wheat
Pinto beans	Black-eyed peas
Red beans	Garbanzo beans
Kidney beans	Kasha
Black beans	Lentils
White beans	Oatmeal
Great Northern beans	Peas
Lima beans	Popcorn, oil-free, air-popped
Snap beans	Potatoes
Beets	Pumpkin
Broadbeans	Rice, brown, wild
Bran	Rice, puffed
Bulgur wheat	Shredded wheat
Corn, white	Soybeans
Corn, yellow	Winter squash, all varieties (is
Corn, sweet	a fibrous carb as well)
Corn grits	Sweet potatoes
Corn tortillas	Yams

Table 14-2

LEAN FIBROUS VEGETABLES

Alfalfa sprouts	Lettuce – Romaine, red leaf,
Asparagus	butter crunch, looseleaf, or
Bamboo shoots	bunching varieties
Beans, green	Mushrooms
Beans, yellow or wax	Mustard greens
Beet greens	Turnips
Broccoli	Spinach
Brussels sprouts	Onions
Cabbage	Peppers, green, red, yellow
Carrots	Peppers, hot
Cauliflower	Pimientos
Broccoflower	Radishes
Celery	Summer squash, all varieties
Collard greens	Tomatoes
Cucumbers	Tomato juice
Eggplant	Turnip greens
Endive	Watercress
Kale	Zucchini
Leeks	

Table 14-3

Low-Sugar Fruits

You may also include another type of carb — low-sugar fruits. These fruits are high in fiber, vitamins, and minerals, yet low in sugar. You get plenty of nutrients, but no uncomfortable, fast release of sugar into your system. Low-sugar fruits make great mid-morning or mid-afternoon snacks.

Limit your consumption of other fruits for the first seven to eight weeks of the eating program. Don't eliminate them altogether, though, since fruit is a very healthy food, loaded with vitamins and minerals.

LOW-SUGAR FRUITS

Granny Smith apples	Cranberries
Green apples	Boysenberries
Strawberries	Green pears
Blackberries	Kiwifruit
Blueberries	

Table 14-4

Essential Fatty Acids

Fatty acids are the chemical building blocks of fat. There are three types, classified according to their hydrogen content: saturated, mono-unsaturated, and polyunsaturated. Only the polyunsaturated fats contain nutrients called "essential fatty acids" or EFAs. These nutrients are linoleic acid, arachidonic acid, and linolenic acid (also one of the omega-3 trio found in fish oils). They are called "essential" because your body can't make them. You have to get them from food, and varying amounts are found in different types of vegetable oils, as well as in seeds, nuts, and green vegetables.

EFAs have several important functions in the body. They're required for normal growth and development and for the healthy functioning of the blood, arteries, and nerves. Also, EFAs are involved in helping with healthy skin and protect your joints. They also assist in the breakdown and metabolism of cholesterol. Without sufficient EFAs, cholesterol can't be properly transported or broken down.

Signs of an EFA deficiency are dry, flaky skin and stiff, painful joints. These symptoms may indicate that your heart, brain, liver, and other internal organs are EFA-deficient as well.

On the Lean Bodies eating program, your daily fat intake should not exceed 10 to 15 percent of your total calories. One of the main reasons for this low ratio is that dietary fat, like simple sugars, is easily converted to body fat. In fact, your body stores calories from fat much more easily than calories from carbohydrates.

To get the right amount of healthy fats, all you have to do is eat 1 to 2 teaspoons of EFAs each day. (Make sure the label states 100% cold-pressed.)

In Table 14-5 is a list of EFAs you may eat on the program.

ESSENTIAL FATTY ACIDS

Borage oil (taken in capsule form - see usage recommendations on bottle) Canola oil Evening Primrose oil (4 to 6 capsules a day) Flaxseed oil	Hain All Blend Safflower oil Salmon oil Soybean oil Sunflower seed oil

Table 14-5

What To Limit

Getting lean and achieving peak health require dedication on your part. So there are foods that should be limited on this program. Later on, when your metabolism runs more effectively, you can re-introduce some of these foods into your lifestyle. For now, limit the following foods the first eight weeks on the program:

• Refined carbohydrates and simple sugars. These easily convert to body fat, plus they can contribute to other ill health effects.

• Fat-free products. Many of these are formulated with refined carbohydrates and sugars to give foods the appearance and consistency of the fattier foods they replace. It's best to limit these products in your diet to keep from eating too many refined carbohydrates. I personally use all the fat-free salad dressings to add flavor, but only sparingly.

• High-fat dairy products. Dairy products such as whole milk, butter, cheeses, or ice cream are high in fat. Like refined carbs, they also can turn into body fat.

However, I'm not saying that these foods are "bad." Using the example of Biblical days again, people living back then needed butter and whole milk to survive. Because of their active, agrarian lifestyles, they had fast metabolisms and, therefore, could handle such foods. But most people today aren't so fortunate. We eat too much saturated fat, and our metabolisms — thanks to sedentary habits — aren't geared up enough to properly process an excess of fat. So we have to limit how much saturated fat we eat. We are "high-tech but low activity."

A final point here: The calcium usually supplied by dairy products can be obtained by dark green leafy vegetables and low-fat dairy products.

• Red meats. Red meat is really a treasure trove of nutrients, including protein, iron, vitamin B12, and more. However, most red meat today is riddled with fat because of the way cattle are purposely fattened. That's why you need to limit red meat in your diet, unless your physician has diagnosed you as anemic.

One of the healthiest red meats, however, is longhorn beef, which is extremely low in fat. Longhorn steers graze in open fields; they're not fattened up for commercial purposes. Back in the 1800s, there were thousands of longhorns, and they almost became extinct because they wouldn't fatten up like other cattle.

But today, the longhorn steer is making a big comeback, and I think you're going to see more grocery stores across the country offering this lean cut of beef.

I'm from Texas and I like a good steak. We offer "Lean Bodies Longhorn Beef," an ultra-lean beef, high in protein and totally natural. We have teamed up with a longhorn producer and can ship directly to your home or restaurant a variety of beef products that meet all Lean Bodies nutritional standards. Call today, 1-800-LEAN.

Other allowable red meats are round steak and tenderloin. Limit your consumption of these to just once a week, however.

• All processed foods. These include canned foods, pre-packaged "quickie foods," and foods containing preservatives.

• Refined and processed pasta and bagels. Many of these foods are nutritious. But the way they are processed today means they are easily changed into sugar, then to body fat. As a Russian trainer friend of mine says: "If you eat noodles, you'll look like noodles."

• High-sugar fruits. All fruits are healthy, full of vitamins, minerals, and fiber. But some fruits — namely bananas, citrus fruits, juices, raisins, and grapes — are higher with the simple sugar fructose. Because of the molecular structure of fructose, it can be converted by the liver into fat, if your metabolism is sub-par. For this reason, the Lean Bodies eating program sticks to low-fructose fruits — Granny Smith apples, strawberries, blueberries, blackberries, and so forth (see Table 14-4 for a complete list). All these have lower amounts of simple sugars in them, and are higher in fiber.

Some remarkable changes will take place in your body as a result of tweaking these foods in your diet. When Dwayne W. cut back on refined pasta, high-sugar fruits, and processed bread — and gradually increased his calories to 5,500 to 6,000 a day, some dramatic changes took place. He peeled his body fat percentage from 10.1 down to 6.2, while increasing his lean mass. Today, Dwayne is a cut-to-the-max 195 pounds — a net gain of 13 pounds of fat-free muscle.

But back to pasta for a moment: Isn't it supposed to be the food of champions? Not if you consider Dwayne's athletic performance. He doesn't load up on pasta, yet competes successfully in triathlons. "I've found I have more energy than ever for my training, plus all through the day."

Eat Throughout The Day

On the Lean Bodies eating program, you eat five or more meals a day. Metabolically, there are excellent reasons for doing so. After a meal, your body begins to burn the food to release energy. This causes a reaction called "thermogenesis," a release of heat from the burning of food. During thermogenesis, the metabolism increases. By eating frequent meals, you keep your metabolism high throughout the day. In other words, if you eat 3,000 calories for the day, you will be leaner if you eat those calories over five or six meals a day as opposed to two meals.

So throughout the day, give your body a constant and steady supply of nutrients to fuel your activities and to be used anabolically. Always eat the most important meal of the day — breakfast. This activates your metabolism for the entire day.

In the Lean Bodies program, we teach you about "special ordering" at restaurants (see *Cliff Sheats Lean Bodies*). I'm happy to report in the Dallas/Fort Worth area there is an upcoming restaurant chain that has designed its menu for your lifestyle. Fresh 'n' Lite Deli and Grill offers great taste, variety and atmosphere. Call them at 214-713-8167 or 817-633-5498.

Building Your Meals

Also, combine foods properly to slow the release of glucose into the bloodstream. If calories are released into the bloodstream too rapidly, as in the case of fast-release foods such as simple sugars and processed foods, the excess can be converted readily into body fat. The proper combination of foods is lean proteins, fibrous vegetables, and starchy carbohydrates.

Each main Lean Bodies meal is made up of:

• A lean protein
• One or two starchy carbohydrates
• A lean, fibrous vegetable

Two "mini" or "mock meals" must be included in your daily menu as well. A mini-meal is approximately one to two ounces of lean protein or low-fat dairy product with 1 cup of a starchy carbohydrate (cooked). A low-sugar fruit can be included, too.

Mock meals are convenient ways to get in your mid-morning and mid-afternoon meals — perfect for an on-the-go lifestyle. They consist of certain supplements, usually eaten along with a starchy carbohydrate. For example:

• A powdered protein/carbohydrate supplement, mixed with water, Crystal Light, or sugar-free Tang (see Appendix C for recommended products).

• A sports nutrition bar (see Appendix C for recommended products).

Don't Go Without Breakfast

No doubt, you've heard the advice, "Breakfast is the most important meal of the day." When you eat a hearty breakfast, you energize yourself for the activities ahead, plus start your metabolism on a roll. But one reason why a lot of people skip breakfast is time. They're too busy in the morning to fix a healthy breakfast. Our solution to your time constraints is The Lean Bodies Quick Breakfast Blend. Simply blend together 8 ounces of non-fat yogurt, 1 cup of raw oats, 1 scoop of a carbohydrate/protein supplement, 1 cup of frozen berries, and enough water to produce a milkshake-like consistency. Our breakfast blend takes just minutes to fix, supplies roughly 700 calories, and gets you off to a great start nutritionally. You have all day to burn those calories!

Counting Calories The Lean Bodies Way

You should try to increase your calories by 100 a week if you're a woman and by 200 a week if you're a man. The first Lean Bodies book is a good guide showing how to do this from week to week.

Calorie-counting doesn't have to be tedious, either. As you plan your meals, you can do it in your head, using the following chart:

QUICK CALORIE COUNT CHART

Food	Quantity	Calories
Lean Protein	1 ounce	25-40
Potato/Sweet Potato	1 ounce	25-30
Grains/Rice/Legumes/Corn	1 cup	180-240
Oatmeal	1 cup	300-390 depending on product (check labels)
Shredded Wheat	Per biscuit	Depends on size (check labels)
Fibrous Vegetables	1 cup	20-50
Low-Sugar Fruits	1 cup or 1 piece	60-80
Non-Fat Yogurt/Skim Milk	1 cup	80-100
Fat	1 teaspoon	45

Table 14-6

What follows are some examples of menus for various caloric intakes. They are divided into Moderate Activity for people who engage in two days of weight training and three days of aerobics, and High Activity for exercisers who perform three or more days of weight training and four or more days of aerobics. The High Activity menus also feature a little extra protein, which you require when exercising at this level. Additional menus can be found in the first Lean Bodies book.

1,500-CALORIE MEAL PLAN

Moderate Activity	High Activity
Breakfast: 3 shredded wheat biscuits 1 cup non-fat yogurt	Breakfast: 8 oz. sweet potato 1 cup skim milk
Mini-Meal: 6 oz. potato 2 oz. tuna	Mini-Meal: 1/2 cup raw oats 4 oz. non-fat yogurt
Lunch: *Corn bread (4 1/2" x 4 1/2") 3 oz. longhorn tenderloin 1 cup green beans	Lunch: 1 cup corn 3 oz. cod 1 cup spinach
Mini-Meal: 3 rice cakes 4 oz. non-fat yogurt	Mock Meal: 2 oz. carbohydrate supplement, mixed with water, Crystal Light or sugar-free Tang
Dinner: 4 oz. sweet potato 3 oz. shrimp 1 cup asparagus	Dinner: 1 cup pinto beans (cooked) 3 oz. longhorn tenderloin 1 cup cauliflower 1 cup carrots
Nutrients: 1,525 calories; 91 grams of protein (24 percent of calories); 249 grams of carbohydrate (67 percent of calories); and 15 grams of fat (9 percent of calories).	Nutrients: 1,555 calories; 96 grams of protein (25 percent of calories); 261 grams of carbohydrate (68 percent of calories); and 11 grams of fat (7 percent of calories).

* Meal option taken from the Lean Bodies Cookbook.

2,000-CALORIE MEAL PLAN

Moderate Activity	High Activity
Breakfast: * 3 pancakes * 1/2 cup raspberry sauce	Breakfast: 10 oz. sweet potato 3 egg whites 1 cup skim milk
Mini-Meal: 2 oz. carbohydrate supplement, mixed with water, Crystal Light or sugar-free Tang 4 rice cakes (Lundberg)	Mock Meal: 2 oz. carbohydrate supplement, mixed with water, Crystal Light or sugar-free Tang
Lunch: 10 oz. potato 4 oz. chicken breast 1 cup asparagus	Lunch: 2 corn tortillas 1 cup brown rice (cooked) 1 cup beans 4 oz. chicken 1/2 cup lettuce & 1/2 cup tomatoes 2 tsp. picante sauce
Mini-Meal: 3 rice cakes 1 Granny Smith apple 8 oz. non-fat yogurt	Mini-Meal: 6 oz. potato 1 tbsp. MCT oil 1 cup green beans
Dinner: 1 cup brown rice (cooked) 4 oz. shrimp 1/2 cup bamboo shoots 1/2 cup water chestnuts 1/2 cup cabbage	Dinner: 6" corn on the cob 4 oz. longhorn tenderloin 1 cup green beans
Nutrients: 2,050 calories; 130 grams of protein (25 percent of calories); 319 grams of carbohydrate (68 percent of calories); and 15 grams of fat (7 percent of calories).	Nutrients: 2,005 calories; 100 grams of protein (20 percent of calories); 354 grams of carbohydrate (71 percent of calories); and 21 grams of fat (9 percent of calories).

* Meal options taken from the *Lean Bodies Cookbook.*

2,500-CALORIE MEAL PLAN

Moderate Activity	High Activity
Breakfast: 8 tbsp. grits 1 tbsp. MCT oil 8 oz. non-fat yogurt	Breakfast: 1 cup raw oats 2 oz. carbohydrate supplement 1 cup berries (your choice) 8 oz. non-fat yogurt
Mini-Meal: 2 corn tortillas 1 cup brown rice (cooked) 2 oz. chicken 1/2 cup broccoli	Mini-Meal: *Corn bread (4 1/2" x 4 1/2") 1 cup skim milk
Lunch: *Corn bread (4 1/2" x 4 1/2") 4 oz. longhorn tenderloin 1 cup green beans	Lunch: *Oven-baked fries (1 medium potato) 1 tbsp. MCT oil 5 oz. salmon 1 cup Romaine lettuce, 1/2 cup tomatoes, 1/2 cup cucumbers
Mini-Meal: 1 sports nutrition bar 3 rice cakes	Mock Meal: 2 oz. carbohydrate supplement, mixed with water, Crystal Light or sugar-free Tang
Dinner: 12 oz. potato 1 tbsp. MCT oil 5 oz. cod 1 cup yellow squash	Dinner: 1 cup corn 5 oz. turkey breast 1 cup cabbage
Nutrients: 2,500 calories; 120 grams of protein (19 percent of calories); 386 grams of carbohydrate (71 percent of calories); and 27 grams of fat (10 percent of calories).	Nutrients: 2,505 calories; 151 grams of protein (24 percent of calories); 381 grams of carbohydrate (66 percent of calories); and 29 grams of fat (10 percent of calories).

* Meal options taken from the *Lean Bodies Cookbook*.

3,000-CALORIE MEAL PLAN

Moderate Activity	High Activity
Breakfast: 1 cup raw oats 10 oz. sweet potato 2 oz. carbohydrate supplement, mixed with water, Crystal Light or sugar-free Tang 8 oz. non-fat yogurt	Breakfast: *4 pancakes (5" diameter) *1/2 cup raspberry sauce 2 oz. carbohydrate supplement, mixed with water, Crystal Light or sugar-free Tang 1 tbsp. MCT oil 3 egg whites
Mini-Meal: 1 sports nutrition bar 1 Granny Smith apple	Mini-Meal: 4 corn tortillas 4 tsp. picante sauce 1 cup brown rice (cooked) 1 cup pinto beans (cooked)
Lunch: 2 cups brown rice (cooked) 1 cup corn 1 tbsp. MCT oil 5 oz. haddock	Lunch: 2 cups corn 6 oz. longhorn tenderloin 2 bell peppers
Mini-Meal: 8 oz. potato 3 oz. tuna	Mock Meal: 2 oz. carbohydrate supplement, mixed with water, Crystal Light or sugar-free Tang
Dinner: 1 cup red beans 1 tbsp. MCT oil 4 oz. longhorn burger 1/2 cup squash	Dinner: 8 oz. sweet potato 6 oz. salmon 1 cup zucchini
Nutrients: 3,015 calories; 150 grams of protein (20 percent of calories); 492 grams of carbohydrate (73 percent of calories); and 24 grams of fat (7 percent of calories).	Nutrients: 3,015 calories; 175 grams of protein (23 percent of calories); 471 grams of carbohydrate (63 percent of calories); and 35 grams of fat (10 percent of calories).

* Meal options taken from the *Lean Bodies Cookbook.*

Your Optimal Fueling Formula

After a few days on the Lean Bodies Workout and eating program, you should figure out your caloric goal: the amount of calories you should build toward, based on your sex and activity level. Here's a formula you can use to calculate the number of calories you will ultimately need each day for optimum fueling and maintenance as your metabolism becomes faster:

BW = Body Weight

BMR = Basal Metabolic Rate (the rate at which calories are burned to fuel the body's basic biological function)

VMA = Voluntary Muscular Activity

SDA = Specific Dynamic Action

BW / 2.2 = BW (*kg) x .9 (for women) = Women's BW kg

BW kg x 24 hrs. = BMR

BMR x .8 (**This number can vary depending on your activity level) = VMA

BMR + VMA = Calories x .1 = SDA

BMR + VMA + SDA = Calories for Optimal Fueling

* A kilogram (kg) equals 2.2 pounds.

** If you are sedentary, use .50 here; moderately active (you exercise 3 to 4 times a week, doing aerobics), .65; and very active, .8 (performing the Lean Bodies Workout as described).

To show you how this formula works, let's suppose you are a very active woman, weighing 57 kg (or 125 pounds). Your calculation would look like this:

125 lbs/2.2 = 57 (kg) x .9 (for women) = Women's 51.3 kg
51.3 kg x 24 hrs. = 1231. 2 (BMR)
1231.2 (BMR) x .8 = 984.96 (VMA)
1231.2 (BMR) + 984.96 (VMA) = 2216.16 (Calories) x .1 =
221.6 (SDA)
1231.2 (BMR) + 984.96 (VMA) + 221.6 (SDA) = 2437.76
Calories for Optimal Fueling

Here's a calculation for a very active man who weighs 79 kg
(or 175 pounds).

79 kg x 24 hrs. = 1896 (BMR)
1896 (BMR) x .8 = 1516.8 (VMA)
1896 (BMR) + 1516.8 (VMA) = 3412.8 (Calories) x .1 = 341
(SDA)
1896 (BMR) + 1516.8 (VMA) + 341 (SDA) = 3754 Calories for
Optimal Fueling

As you become more active, always remember to increase
your calories to match your level of training. In my opinion, too
many people are working out in an undernourished state, and this
cancels out the positive effects of exercise on the body.

Water

Don't ignore the thirst signal, especially while working out.
Drinking adequate water has some real benefits when you're trying to get lean.

First, water and fluids help your body store glycogen for use
later as energy.

Second, water assists your kidneys in effectively removing waste products from your system.

Third, it also serves as a medium for every enzymatic and chemical reaction in the body, including the digestion and fat-burning, and it transports nutrients and oxygen to every cell in the body.

More than 75 percent of your body is made up of water. You can survive without food for days, but, without water, dehydration begins in just a few hours. Next to oxygen, water is the substance most important for life.

I recommend that you drink 8 to 10 large glasses of water every day. One of the best sources is spring water because of its mineral content or carbon pressed filtered water. The latter is an inexpensive product that effectively removes chemicals from water but preserves the mineral content.

Planned Deviations:
A Great Benefit Of A Faster Metabolism

Ever hear a little voice in your head whispering "just this once ..."?

"Just this once have an ice cream sundae ... a pizza ... some chips and dip."

We're free to make that choice. But after we do, that choice seizes control of us. We feel guilty. We feel like a failure. We're ready to throw in the towel.

What if you do have a tiny cheat? First of all, stop berating yourself. Start back on the plan at your very next meal. It may comfort you to know that because your metabolism is faster by now, your body can handle that cheat better than ever. So don't despair.

On most diets, that cheat would have been more easily converted to body fat. That's because the body thinks it's starving, so the special fat storage enzyme I mentioned earlier goes to work, telling your body to stockpile fat once it's fed again.

Before you were on the Lean Bodies eating program, there might have been a time in your dieting life when every goody seemed to turn right into body fat, no matter how small the portion. You probably ate a lot of goodies, especially after falling off the "diet wagon." On Lean Bodies, there's no wagon to fall off of. In the first place, you're eating more calories and more food. You're not hungry, so you don't feel like "pigging out."

Every once in a while, you may eat foods that aren't on the program. But metabolically, now you can handle it. As you start experiencing how well your body uses food, you won't feel guilty about eating foods that are forbidden on most diets. Remember, too, that exercise is a key component of weight control because it expends calories for energy — so maintain your level of activity.

I recommend to people that they practice something I call a "planned deviation." Simply put, this means planning to eat a treat one day a week only — without eating on impulse. Impulsive eating leads to more impulsive eating, not to mention a pile of guilt. When you plan your deviations, you give yourself permission to eat, and there's no guilt.

You can't go on planned cheats every day, however. That would defeat your goal of losing body fat and gaining lean mass. While keeping your calories up, you must continue to eat lean proteins, starchy carbohydrates, lean, fibrous vegetables, and essential fatty acids — in the amounts suggested on the Lean Bodies eating program.

15

Say Goodbye To Fatigue

CHAPTER FIFTEEN

MELISSA P. USED TO FEEL SO DRAGGED OUT that even a minimal amount of physical effort was draining. She felt chronically tired, experienced shortness of breath, and was overweight. To Melissa, following a regular exercise program was the impossible dream. But she decided to give Lean Bodies a try anyway. Here's what happened, in her own words:

"In just three short weeks, I had a higher energy level. The eight-week exercise program, combined with the suggested meal plans, resulted in physical improvements. In five weeks, I decreased my dress size by one size. All my thanks go to Lean Bodies."

We meet so many people like Melissa who come to Lean Bodies tuckered out and run-down. A common complaint is "I have no energy." But in a matter of weeks, after starting the program, they're transformed, ready to take on the world, run a marathon.

What's going on here? To answer that question, let's explore the reasons for fatigue — and the solutions in terms of nutrition and exercise.

CP Depletion

If you recall, CP (creatine phosphate) is the tiny energy supply available in muscles to rebuild ATP and help maintain your stores of ATP. Studies have shown that fatigue corresponds with the depletion of CP during repeated intense muscular contractions.[1] When CP is emptied, it's difficult for the body to quickly replenish ATP. ATP levels fall off, and fatigue sets in.

You can prevent CP depletion in two ways. First, pace yourself when you begin exercising. In other words, don't run as fast as you can the first leg of your aerobic workout. Likewise, don't start lifting the heaviest weight for the highest number of repetitions the minute you start your weight training workout. Regulate your training pace to avoid premature fatigue, while still gradually building your intensity. That way, you'll allow your body to more efficiently use ATP and CP for the duration of your exercise session.

Second, if you would like, try supplementation with creatine monohydrate. This builds levels of creatine in the muscle to improve performance, particularly in weight training. Creatine supplementation is covered in Chapter 18. Be sure to review the information to learn how to prevent fatigue with this supplement.

Glycogen Depletion

Exercise can quickly deplete glycogen, a source of energy for the working muscles. The more intense your activity, the faster glycogen is depleted. If you run sprints, for example, muscle glycogen is used up 35 to 40 times faster than if you just walk.[2]

Following a diet in which at least 65 percent of the total calories come from carbohydrates will keep your muscles well-supplied with glycogen when you need it. As the Lean Bodies eating program recommends, most of these carbs should be complex, starchy carbohydrates. This is the real "gasoline" that powers you for daily activity and exercise.

On the Lean Bodies eating program, you're eating throughout the day. This helps stabilize your blood sugar for a slow, enduring release of energy. What's more, the mix of foods you're eating is specially designed to elevate energy. The combination of lean protein and high-fiber vegetables is digested slowly. There's an even release of energy as a result.

It's well-known that more muscle — accompanied by proper recovery and ample carbs — stores a lot more glycogen than untrained muscle. A point of proof: When distance runners, for example, took a few days off from training and ate a carb-rich diet, their muscles stockpiled twice as much glycogen as inactive people who ate the same diet.[3] So the better trained you are, the better your muscles store energy-yielding glycogen.

Undereating And Overexercising

The most common "energy crisis" I see among people is undereating and overexercising — that is, doing hours of exercise each week while subsisting on low-calorie diets of 1,100 to 1,200 calories a day. Those practices will sap your energy in a hurry, plus keep your body in a state of tissue breakdown (catabolism). Low-calorie dieting can also deplete your stores of iron, a mineral involved in energy production. (I cover the topic of iron and fatigue in Chapter 21.)

Michelle D. is a good example of someone who used to overexercise and undereat. She taught two aerobics classes a day, hardly ate anything, yet still couldn't lose body fat. Her metabolism had ground to a halt.

Once on the Lean Bodies eating program, Michelle began fueling herself every two to three hours — and adding more protein to her diet, as suggested. "This approach gave me more energy than I had ever had and made my workouts much easier."

Michelle was able to compete in her first marathon recently. Not only that, she's lost 4 percent body fat!

Of course, at various times very low-calorie diets have been the rage, and millions of people have participated in them, since these regimens promise weight losses of 10 or more pounds a week. These diets are deficient in key nutrients, and many people go on them without medical supervision. In their heyday, such diets resulted in about 60 deaths, many of which were attributed to loss of lean tissue, particularly heart muscle.[4]

By eating too few calories, you're not fueling your body properly. Lack of fuel throws everything out of whack — even your mental processes. Your brain needs a steady supply of blood sugar to operate. Without it, you can't think clearly. You even feel drowsy. Your motivation to continue the diet suffers. At that point, you are likely to gorge on stuff you shouldn't, like high-fat, sugary foods.

The other issue is this: Low-calorie dieting combined with exercise makes your metabolic rate plummet. Your body simply can't generate energy when it's in a calorie-deficient state created by undereating and overexercising. You have to reach the correct balance, and that includes increasing calories from the right kind of food.

Overtraining

Overtraining occurs when you exercise so much and so hard that your body can't properly recover. Consequently, it starts breaking down more tissue than it builds. The first sign of overtraining is a drop in performance. You can't lift as much weight, run as fast or as long, walk without getting winded.

Other symptoms include fatigue, weight loss, decrease in

appetite, sleep problems, elevated resting heart rate, and depressed immune function that can lead to colds and infection.

One of America's best-known training experts, John Parrillo, has put a new spin on overtraining. He calls it "under-nutrition" — not taking in enough nutrients in the form of food and supplements to assist your body in rebuilding itself after workouts.

While many experts would say the problem is more complex than that, I do agree with John. Nutrition and adequate rest are the two best ways to treat overtraining. Particular attention must be paid to carbohydrate and protein intake. Carbohydrates replenish your body's energy reserves, plus supply nutrients called "antioxidants" (see Chapter 17) that stimulate recovery processes. Protein provides the amino acids required to repair and build muscle tissue in the aftermath of exercise.

Metabolic By-Products Of Exercise

In brief bursts of muscular effort like weight training, lactic acid builds up in the muscle, creating the sensation known as "the burn." You feel fatigued and can no longer continue muscular contractions, so you rest. During your rest periods, this sensation subsides, and you can resume exercise.

It's not the lactic acid buildup, per se, that causes fatigue but rather the metabolic by-products, namely hydrogen ions and lactate, that it produces. These create a more acidic environment in the muscles — a condition that disrupts cellular energy production and muscular contraction.

The ability to stall this type of fatigue comes with training experience. In other words, the more trained your muscles are, the longer it will take for lactic acid to accumulate in them, thereby postponing the buildup of these metabolic by-products.

Other Causes Of Fatigue

The causes of fatigue discussed thus far involve muscle metabolism — the conversion of nutrients into energy inside muscle cells. When nutrients are in short supply, your body seems to compensate by making you feel like you need a nap. But there may be more to fatigue than just muscular metabolism. Scientists are beginning to think that certain potent brain chemicals play a role, too.

One of these is serotonin, a "neurotransmitter." Neurotransmitters send nerve impulses between nerve cells and other cells. Serotonin is one of more than 40 neurotransmitters that have been identified in the body. Among other functions, serotonin seems to regulate drowsiness.

The landmark work in this area of exercise fatigue has been conducted by Eric Newsholme, Ph. D., at Oxford University, who has extensively researched serotonin. Basically, the more serotonin your brain releases, the drowsier you feel. Dr. Newsholme calls this the "central nervous system hypothesis" of fatigue.[5]

Exercising for a long time hikes blood levels of the amino acid tryptophan, which the brain changes into serotonin. If you could somehow limit the release of serotonin, then maybe you'd get less fatigued after exercise and possibly extend your endurance.

One way to do that would be to keep tryptophan from reaching the brain. Dr. Newsholme speculated that getting more branched-chain amino acids (BCAAs) into the blood would do just that. The reason? BCAAs vie with tryptophan for entry to the brain. Higher levels of BCAAs would in effect block tryptophan from reaching the brain and being converted into serotonin.

Dr. Newsholme put his theory to the test by concocting a sports drink loaded with BCAAs and giving it to athletes prior to competition. The results of two of his experiments were featured in the August 1994 issue of *Runner's World* magazine. In one study, BCAA-supplemented soccer players scored better on a mental functioning test after a match than before it.

In the other — a study of marathon runners — slower BCAA-supplemented runners bettered their time by five or six minutes. In the *Runner's World* article, Newsholme explained that slower, less fit runners probably release more free fatty acids, which tend to elevate tryptophan. So it stands to reason that the BCAAs would go to work more readily when there's a lot of tryptophan around.

I was intrigued by this research, particularly since I supplement with BCAAs. From personal experience, I feel that they do help my energy levels, plus provide insurance that I'm getting the amino acids I need to support muscle growth and repair.

Elsewhere, research in the United States has shown that sports drinks containing carbohydrates keep tryptophan levels under wraps during exercise, thus limiting increases in serotonin. So it looks like carb supplements not only replace glycogen and delay muscle fatigue, they also reduce central nervous system fatigue.

The fascinating research into brain chemicals and exercise continues, and I suspect that much more will be learned in the future about manipulating serotonin and other neurotransmitters for better performance.

16

My Two-Week Fat-Burning Blitz

SOMETIMES, your body needs an extra nudge to burn more fat. My Two-Week Fat-Burning Blitz is one sure way. Begin now, and you'll start seeing results in only a few days.

The best thing about this plan is that you don't have to deprive yourself of food. There's no crash dieting on 800 calories a day or less. You actually get to eat more food — not less — and knock off body fat in the process.

There's no guesswork involved either. I tell you what to do each day for two weeks. It's easy to follow, and best of all, it works. All you have to do is follow my exact instructions for meals and exercise each day of the plan. Then watch the fat melt off … in just two weeks.

Now, a few points about how the blitz works:

Manipulate Your Carbohydrate Calories To Maximize Fat-Burning

You'll follow the same menu plan as you have followed up to now, but with an important exception. Four times a week, you'll eliminate starchy carbohydrates from your evening meal. In other words, no starchy carbs after 3 p.m. in the afternoon. There are three reasons for this.

Reason one: By reducing your carbohydrate consumption, you inhibit the release of the hormone insulin. One of insulin's jobs is to promote fat storage. Inhibiting the secretion of insulin triggers glucagon, a hormone that helps unlock fat stores.

Reason two: When starchy carbohydrates are dropped at night, fewer stored carbohydrates (glycogen) are available for energy the next morning. In the absence of glycogen, your body starts burning fatty acids (stored body fat) for energy when you exercise aerobically before breakfast, as the plan recommends. Fat loss is accelerated as a result.

Reason three: When you eat starchy carbohydrates at breakfast and lunch, they are efficiently converted into glycogen for storage in the muscles — and are less likely to be converted to fat.

You may feel slightly less energetic from the exclusion of starchy carbohydrates. If this happens to you, compensate by eating more of these carbohydrates all through the day (except at dinner time). It also helps to supplement with MCT oil, taken with food in the afternoon, with mock meals, and in the evening. Used this way, MCT oil acts as a pure energy source because it is absorbed like a carbohydrate; it spares glycogen; it helps your body enter a fat-burning mode; and it helps speed up your metabolism. For more information on how MCT oil works, see Chapter 20.

Use My Proven Fat-Burning Exercise Techniques

My blitz incorporates two important fat-burning techniques that were explained in Chapter 11: pre-breakfast aerobics and post-weight training aerobics. In both cases, you are in a glycogen-needy state. Theoretically, your body is forced to draw on its own stored fat for fuel in the absence of enough glycogen for energy. This accelerates fat-burning. We've seen this occur among Lean Bodies clients who perform pre-breakfast or post-weight training aerobics.

You have two options, depending on your schedule. In Option #1, you will exercise aerobically six mornings a week (pre-breakfast) for 45 minutes each time. In Option #2, you do the same, but only three mornings a week. You get your other three sessions in after your weight training workout.

Double Up On Your Aerobics

In both options, I recommend 45 minutes of aerobics in the evening on non-weight training days (30 minutes on weight-training days). This does two things: First, it causes further glycogen depletion, so that in the morning, your body starts immediately deducting fat from storage. Second, evening aerobics crank up your metabolic rate at a time when it tends to drop (during sleep). Remember, vigorous exercise boosts metabolism long after you've finished exercising. Also, the greater the intensity of exercise, the greater the metabolic after-effect.

Weight Train Using A Split Routine

That way, you can get in one more calorie-burning workout each week, plus concentrate on trouble spots that need extra work. If your lower body needs more reshaping, for example, then work it twice a week and your upper body once a week. See the split routines in Chapter 12 for workouts that best suit your goals.

Earning Your Right To Do The Blitz

There's one catch to all of this: You can start the blitz only if you've followed the eight-week Lean Bodies Workout to the letter. It takes eight weeks to become a better metabolizer and to condition your body for intense aerobic and weight training workouts. If you jump into the blitz without this preparation, you won't get the results you're after, and you could risk hurting yourself. Also, don't stay on this blitz longer than two weeks.

So as long as you've completed the eight-week workout, you're ready to try the blitz. Put it all together with the blitz calendar that follows. Stick to it, and see a firmer, fitter body in no time at all!

Reports From Lean Bodies Who Completed The Blitz

As soon as we introduced the Two-Week Fat-Burning Blitz as part of the Lean Bodies program, people were enthusiastic and eager to try it. Here are just a handful of comments (along with portions of their records) that have come to me from Lean Bodies who successfully finished the blitz.

"I used the blitz to get ready for my 25th high school reunion, and I was amazed by the fast results. The first week, I had noticeably more muscle definition, and by the end of the two-week period, I had lost three more pounds. Last year, I tried a popular 14-day crash diet to get ready for a beach vacation, and it was a dismal failure. I lost no weight and felt miserable in my bathing suit. By contrast, I was able to eat approximately 2,000 calories a day on the two-week blitz and get in superb physical condition — better than I've looked in years. At my reunion, I won an award — Least Recognizable Female. I took it as a compliment, since I was much heavier 25 years ago." (Margaret R.)

Sample Daily Report (Margaret R.)

Meal	Foods
Breakfast:	1 cup picante vegetable juice; 1/2 serving oatmeal; 1/2 serving bran; 2 egg whites; 1/2 cup skim milk
Mock Meal:	1 Parrillo Supplement Bar
Lunch:	1 1/4 cup oysters; 1 cup corn; 1 baked potato; 1 cup Romaine lettuce; 1 cup salad vegetables
Mock Meal:	Protein shake
Dinner:	5 oz. lean round steak; 1 onion; 2 cups mixed salad vegetables
Workout:	Split routine, followed by 45 minutes of aerobics

"I followed Option #1. Plus, I added another day of weight training to my exercise schedule. My routine was organized as follows: chest/back/triceps twice a week; shoulders/biceps/legs twice a week. I also biked, elevating my heart rate to 160 to 165, and ran, with an exercising heart rate of 140 to 160. For variety, I played a lot of full-court basketball.

"Where nutrition is concerned, I eliminated starchy carbohydrates at night, while eating more of them during the day. My calories ranged from 4,200 to 5,000 a day.

"After just a few days on the blitz, I definitely showed a leaner physique, with no loss of energy. By the end of the blitz, I lost body fat and gained muscle." (Dwayne W.)

Sample Daily Report (Dwayne W.)

Meal	Foods
Breakfast:	2 cups rolled oats (dry); 8 oz. non-fat yogurt; 6 egg whites; 4 scoops carbohydrate/protein powder
Mini-Meal #1:	Lean Bodies waffle with strawberry puree (see *Lean Bodies Cookbook* for recipe); 6 egg white omelette; fluid-electrolyte drink
Mini-Meal #2:	Apple muffins (see *Lean Bodies Cookbook* for recipe); corn tortilla; 4 egg whites; 1 cup rice (cooked)
Lunch:	5 oz. skinless chicken breast; 1 1/2 cups green beans; 16 oz. sweet potato
Mock Meal:	Parrillo Supplement Bar; carbohydrate/protein supplement shake (4 scoops carbohydrate/protein powder)
Dinner:	Lean Bodies turkey loaf (see *Lean Bodies Cookbook* for recipe); 1 1/2 cups green beans; 2 cups corn
Workout:	4-day split routine: Day 1: chest/back/triceps; Day 2: shoulders, biceps, legs; biking, running, full-court basketball

"When I first looked at the Two-Week Fat-Burning Blitz, I was overwhelmed. I thought: 'I can't do it!' But I just took one step at a time. My calories averaged between 2,200 and 2,500 a day. I was surprised that I had so much energy to do the exercise routines. And I was thrilled with the muscular definition the blitz produced." (Kathy S.)

Sample Daily Report (Kathy S.)

Meal	Foods
Early morning mini-meal:	2 scoops carbohydrate/protein powder mixed in 1 cup skim milk
Breakfast:	1 cup raw oats with 2 scoops carbohydrate/protein powder; 1/2 cup skim milk
Mock Meal:	1 Parrillo Supplement Bar; 1 cup non-fat yogurt
Lunch:	4 oz. crispy baked chicken (See *Lean Bodies Cookbook* for recipe); 10 oz. baked potato with MCT oil and Molly McButter; 1 cup salad vegetables
Mini-Meal:	3 shredded wheat biscuits; 2 scoops carbohydrate/protein powder mixed in 1 cup skim milk
Dinner:	6 egg whites scrambled with 1/2 cup mushrooms and 1/2 cup chopped tomatoes; 1 1/2 cup salad vegetables
Workout:	Weight training three times a week; 45 minutes of morning aerobics, and 30 minutes of aerobics in the evening

"I used a number of intensity-builders in my workouts, including a split weight training routine and brief rest periods (approximately 30 seconds) between chest, back, frontal thigh, and hamstring exercise sets; 15 to 20 second rest periods between calf exercise sets. My weight training workout was very aerobic, and I was able to elevate my heart rate to 120 to 160 beats a minute while training.

"For aerobics, I did a form of interval training (15-minute bike sprints on a 10-speed, immediately followed by 13, 30-yard running sprints. I walked back to the starting point to begin the next sprint.). My calories averaged between 3,000 and 3,500 a day. The combination of increased calories and higher intensity caused me to lean out considerably." (Wes C.)

Sample Daily Report (Wes C.)

Meal	Foods
Breakfast:	2 1/2 cups rolled oats (dry); 4 scoops protein powder
Mock Meal:	1 Parrillo Supplement Bar
Lunch:	7 1/2 oz. skinless chicken; 2 cups long-grain white rice (cooked); 1 cup black beans
Mock Meal:	Carbohydrate/protein supplement shake (2 scoops carbohydrate/protein powder)
Dinner:	8 oz. longhorn beef; 2 cups broccoli
Workout:	Three days on/one day off split routine (Day 1: chest and back; Day 2: thighs and calves; Day 3: arms and shoulders; Day 4: rest). For aerobics: two 30-minute sessions, alternating between treadmills, walking and recumbent cycling; plus two high-intensity aerobic workouts (sprints) done in an interval-type style

"The results we've seen from the Two-Week Fat-Burning Blitz convinced me that I had to get in the act, too! On the blitz, I worked out on a four-day-a-week split routine and followed the framework of Option #2 (weight training followed by approximately 30 minutes of aerobics. I also performed 45 minutes of aerobics after dinner.

"The first week, I eliminated starchy carbohydrates three nights, and the second week, a little more, depending on my energy levels. On average, my calories ranged from 3,000 to 3,500 a day. I lost body fat and am showing more striations on my upper body, especially in my midsection. (Cliff S.)

Sample Daily Report (Cliff S.)

Meal	Foods
Breakfast:	2 cups Shiloh rolled oats (dry); 8 oz. non-fat yogurt; 1 medium Granny Smith apple; 1 oz. carbohydrate/protein supplement (blender)
Mini-Meal:	1 1/4 cups Shiloh rolled oats (dry); 1 oz. carbohydrate/protein supplement
Lunch:	5 oz. skinless chicken; 1/2 cups long-grain white rice (cooked); 1/2 cup onions (steamed)
Mock Meal:	1/2 cup pinto beans (cooked); 8 corn tortillas; 1/2 cup green pepper (raw); 1 Parrillo Supplement Bar
Dinner:	8 oz. skinless chicken breast; 2 1/2 cups broccoli; 1 1/4 cup black-eyed cowpeas; 1/2 cup string beans (boiled); 2 tbsp. fat-free salad dressing
Workout:	4-day split routine; post-weight training aerobics (30 minutes); evening aerobics (45 minutes)

OPTION #1

MONDAY	TUESDAY	WEDNESDAY	THURSDAY	FRIDAY	SATURDAY	SUNDAY
• 45 minutes of aerobics before breakfast • Eliminate starchy carbs from breakfast • Weight training workout • Include starchy carbs at dinner • After-dinner aerobics for 30 minutes	• 45 minutes of aerobics before breakfast • Eliminate starchy carbs from dinner • Include starchy carbs at dinner • After-dinner aerobics for 30 minutes	• 45 minutes of aerobics before breakfast • Eliminate starchy carbs from dinner • Include starchy carbs at dinner • After-dinner aerobics for 45 minutes	• 45 minutes of aerobics before breakfast • Eliminate starchy carbs from dinner • Include starchy carbs at dinner • After-dinner aerobics for 30 minutes	• 45 minutes of aerobics before breakfast • Eliminate starchy carbs from dinner • Include starchy carbs at dinner • After-dinner aerobics for 45 minutes	• 45 minutes of aerobics before breakfast • Eliminate starchy carbs from dinner • After-dinner aerobics for 45 minutes	• Off • Eliminate starchy carbs from dinner

MONDAY	TUESDAY	WEDNESDAY	THURSDAY	FRIDAY	SATURDAY	SUNDAY
• 45 minutes of aerobics before breakfast • Eliminate starchy carbs from dinner • Weight training workout • Include starchy carbs at dinner • After-dinner aerobics for 45 minutes	• 45 minutes of aerobics before breakfast • Eliminate starchy carbs from dinner • Include starchy carbs at dinner • After-dinner aerobics for 30 minutes	• 45 minutes of aerobics before breakfast • Eliminate starchy carbs from dinner • Include starchy carbs at dinner • After-dinner aerobics for 45 minutes	• 45 minutes of aerobics before breakfast • Eliminate starchy carbs from dinner • Include starchy carbs at dinner • After-dinner aerobics for 30 minutes	• 45 minutes of aerobics before breakfast • Eliminate starchy carbs from dinner • Include starchy carbs at dinner • After-dinner aerobics for 45 minutes	• 45 minutes of aerobics before breakfast • Eliminate starchy carbs from dinner • After-dinner aerobics for 45 minutes	• Off • Eliminate starchy carbs from dinner

OPTION #2

MONDAY	TUESDAY	WEDNESDAY	THURSDAY	FRIDAY	SATURDAY	SUNDAY
• Eat breakfast • Weight training workout* followed by 30 minutes of aerobics • Include starchy carbs at dinner • After-dinner aerobics for 45 minutes	• 45 minutes of aerobics before breakfast • Eliminate starchy carbs from dinner • Include starchy carbs at dinner • After-dinner aerobics for 30 minutes	• Eat breakfast • Weight training workout* followed by 30 minutes of aerobics • Include starchy carbs at dinner • After-dinner aerobics for 45 minutes	• 45 minutes of aerobics before breakfast • Eliminate starchy carbs from dinner • Include starchy carbs at dinner • After-dinner aerobics for 30 minutes	• Eat breakfast • Weight training workout* followed by 30 minutes of aerobics • Include starchy carbs at dinner • After-dinner aerobics for 45 minutes	• 45 minutes of aerobics before breakfast • Eliminate starchy carbs from dinner • After-dinner aerobics for 45 minutes	• Off • Eliminate starchy carbs from dinner

MONDAY	TUESDAY	WEDNESDAY	THURSDAY	FRIDAY	SATURDAY	SUNDAY
• Eat breakfast • Weight training workout* followed by 30 minutes of aerobics • Include starchy carbs at dinner • After-dinner aerobics for 30 minutes	• 45 minutes of aerobics before breakfast • Eliminate starchy carbs from dinner • Include starchy carbs at dinner • After-dinner aerobics for 30 minutes	• Eat breakfast • Weight training workout* followed by 30 minutes of aerobics • Include starchy carbs at dinner • After-dinner aerobics for 30 minutes	• 45 minutes of aerobics before breakfast • Eliminate starchy carbs from dinner • Include starchy carbs at dinner • After-dinner aerobics for 30 minutes	• Eat breakfast • Weight training workout* followed by 30 minutes of aerobics • Include starchy carbs at dinner • After-dinner aerobics for 30 minutes	• 45 minutes of aerobics before breakfast • Eliminate starchy carbs from dinner • After-dinner aerobics for 45 minutes	• Off • Eliminate starchy carbs from dinner

*All weight training workouts on the Two-Week Fat-Burning Blitz are performed as split routines. You may switch the weight training/aerobic session to other dinner if it fits your schedule better. Perform your other aerobic session before breakfast.

Part IV

High-Test Supplements For The Lean Bodies Workout

17

CHAPTER SEVENTEEN

Nutrient Protectors

THE EXERCISING BODY is a nutrient-needy body! As you increase your exercise intensity on the Lean Bodies Workout, you'll need more nutrients for fuel, growth and maintenance, and recovery. That's why you should look into nutritional supplementation, in addition to increasing your calories.

Unlike some nutritionists, I do believe in supplements, but I don't advise going overboard and spending your paycheck to fill your medicine cabinet with pills and quick fixes. The main reason why we all need to supplement has to do with soil depletion. Because of environmental problems and modern farming methods, our soil no longer has ample nutrients, and that means our foods are becoming increasingly nutrient-poor as well. So we have to get protection somewhere, and supplements are our best bet.

There are several classes of protective nutrients with which you may need to consider supplementing your diet: antioxidants, carotenoids (another type of antioxidant), electrolytes, calcium, and chondroprotective agents. Let's begin with antioxidants.

Antioxidants

Antioxidants are nutrients that fight free radicals — nasty little molecules that destroy cells. Your body creates free radicals every time you breathe, eat a meal, react to stress, bask in the sun, or exercise. Yes, exercise!

Free radicals contain one or more unpaired and unstable electrons. Highly reactive, free radicals roam the body unchecked, grabbing electrons of other molecules and claiming them as their own. The process of pairing up with molecules for electrons is called "cellular oxidation." Cellular oxidation is similar to the reaction that rusts metal or turns oils rancid, and it's just as damaging to the body.

If free radicals aren't squelched, a process called "lipid peroxidation" takes over. In a domino-like series of chemical reactions, free radicals hook up with fatty acids in the body to form substances called "peroxides." Peroxides attack cell membranes, setting off a chain reaction that creates many more free radicals. Pits form in cell membranes, allowing harmful bacteria, viruses, and other disease-causing agents to gain entry into cells. Other structures such as body proteins, DNA (the genetic material inside cells), and cartilage can be attacked by free radicals and damaged, too.

What Are Antioxidants?

Certain nutrients called antioxidants help keep free radicals at bay and reduce lipid peroxidation. Vitamin C, vitamin E, and beta carotene are the chief vitamin antioxidants. The antioxidant minerals include selenium, zinc, copper, and manganese. They're involved synergistically in the formation and activity of antioxidant enzymes, substances that inactivate free radicals.

Research has shown that antioxidants have the power to prevent or minimize free radical damage associated with certain diseases, including cancer, cardiovascular disease, arthritis, and cataracts.

Exercise And Antioxidants

As I mentioned previously, exercise is among the factors that can cause the formation of free radicals. One reason is that exercise places such a high demand on the oxidative energy system, producing a condition known as "oxidative stress."[1] It is caused by lipid peroxidation and creates a situation in which free radicals outnumber antioxidants. Scientists can measure oxidative stress in an athlete or exerciser by identifying by-products of lipid peroxidation in expired air samples, muscle biopsies, or in urine.

Antioxidants are important nutrients for exercisers since they can fend off exercise-generated free radicals. All antioxidants have this capability, but vitamin E is especially protective. Known as a natural and effective antioxidant, vitamin E plays a role in the health of skeletal muscle, where it prevents free radicals from attacking cell membranes and causing lipid peroxidation. In essence, vitamin E protects your muscles.

In one study, 21 men (nine were aged 22 to 29, and twelve were 55 to 74) received either 800 IU of vitamin E or placebo daily. After 48 days, they exercised at 75 percent of their maximum heart rate by running for 45 minutes on an incline treadmill. By taking muscle biopsies and analyzing urine, the researchers measured the degree of lipid peroxidation in all the men and found that it was greatly reduced among those who had taken the supplements. What this indicates is that vitamin E appears to protect against exercise-induced oxidative stress.[2]

As noted previously, free radicals can damage DNA, the genetic material inside cells. It appears, however, that vitamin E supplementation may reverse this damage. A case in point: A recent study in Germany looked into the effects of supplementation on DNA damage as a result of exercise. Volunteers ran on a treadmill until they were exhausted. The researchers took blood samples from the volunteers before and 24 hours after the run. They could clearly see DNA strand breakage — an indication of DNA damage.

When the volunteers took a supplement of vitamin E (1,200 IU daily) for 14 days prior to a run, DNA damage was significantly less. In four out of five volunteers, supplementation completely prevented DNA damage.[3]

Vitamin C may hold some promise for exercisers, too. Scientists from the University of Birmingham in England have proof that vitamin C may help your muscles recover faster from intense exercise. Over a three-week experimental period, they had students supplement their diets with either 400 mg of vitamin C, 400 IU of vitamin E, or a placebo. Each group exercised strenuously for 60 minutes, stepping up and down on a knee-high box at an average rate of 24 steps a minute.

In follow-up tests, the scientists found that the vitamin C-supplemented exercisers recovered best of all. They had less muscle soreness during the 24-hour follow-up period. Plus, they regained 85 percent of their leg strength (the other groups had regained only 75 percent).

How exactly did vitamin C make the difference? The scientists raised two possibilities: First, vitamin C may have neutralized free radicals, thus preventing damage to cell membranes during exercise. Second, it may have kept vitamin E stores intact, further protecting muscles from the stress of exercise.[4]

The mineral selenium is an important member of the antioxidant defense team, too. Its chief role is in the formation of the antioxidant enzyme known as glutathione peroxidase. This enzyme detoxifies cancer-causing agents and can turn free radicals into water.

Selenium also protects cell membranes from free radical attack, possibly by reducing lipid peroxides. In one study, 33 swimmers supplemented with selenium (150 mcg) for two weeks. Following exercise, their levels of peroxides were significantly reduced, and levels of glutathione were protected. These findings indicate that selenium enhances and protects the antioxidant status of athletes.[5]

Many other studies have turned up similar findings: that vitamin E and other antioxidants guard against free radical damage caused by exercise. Based on such compelling evidence, these nutrients should definitely be part of your nutritional arsenal. But be sure you're eating properly first. Supplements should complement your eating program.

Supplementing With Antioxidants

If you had to take only one supplement, I advise supplementing with an antioxidant formula. We have found that many antioxidant supplements have a full range of all essential nutrients; others are formulated with antioxidants only. For best results, choose a "co-natural" formulation that contains all the antioxidants, in addition to a base formula of other nutrients. If you feel as though you need additional antioxidants such as vitamin C or vitamin E, you can take them in addition to your antioxidant supplement.

Table 17-1 lists the antioxidant nutrients and their function in exercise performance. Whatever supplement you decide to take, be sure to talk to your doctor first.

Getting Your Antioxidants To Work Better

If you want to squeeze every bit of nutrient power from your antioxidants, here are some tips to help you:

• Take your vitamin C in divided doses. If you've decided to supplement with extra vitamin C, don't take it all at once. It's been estimated that if you take 100 mg at a time, a higher percentage will be absorbed. But taking 1,000 mg at once cuts absorption by as much as half. So the lower the dose, the better the absorption. Another option is to choose a time-release vitamin C formula.

• Vitamins E, D, and A are fat-soluble vitamins. They're absorbed in the presence of fat, so it's best to take them with foods containing a bit of fat, such as skim milk, a chicken breast, or salad with low-fat dressing. Having some fat in your intestine triggers the secretion of digestive enzymes that promote the absorption of fat-soluble vitamins. Without some dietary fat, these vitamins can sail right through your system without being well-absorbed.

Antioxidant Nutrients In Performance

Antioxidant	Performance-Related Function	Food Sources	*General Usage Guidelines
Beta Carotene	Inhibits a destructive free radical known as singlet oxygen, which can cause cancer; may work in concert with other antioxidants to prevent oxidative stress	Yellow and orange vegetables and fruits	15,000 IU to 50,000 IU daily
Vitamin C	Helps convert certain free radicals into less reactive molecules; may work	Berries, citrus fruits, vegetables	.5 gram to 2 grams daily

continued on page 232

Antioxidant	Performance-Related Function	Food Sources	*General Usage Guidelines
	in concert with other antioxidants to prevent oxidative stress		
Vitamin E	Reduces oxidative damage caused by exercise; protects heart health	Vegetable oils, whole grains	200 IU to 800 IU daily
Selenium	Required to make antioxidant enzymes; reduces oxidative damage caused by exercise; may prevent fatigue and promote recovery	Whole grains, chicken, seafood, broccoli, onions, garlic	70 μg for men; 55 μg for women
Zinc	Required to make antioxidant enzymes	Animal foods, whole grains, oysters	15 mg for men; 12 mg for women
Copper	Required to make antioxidant enzymes; involved in the formation of hemoglobin and red blood cells by helping with iron absorption	Whole grains, shellfish, eggs, legumes, and green leafy vegetables	2 mg.
Manganese	Required to make antioxidant enzymes	Whole grains, vegetables	5 mg a day

Table 17-1

* *Check with your physician for recommended dosages of nutrients.*

Carotenoids

While antioxidants have grabbed their share of attention in nutrition, there's a new kid on the block — carotenoids, a kind of super-antioxidant now making news. Carotenoids are components of fruits and vegetables that have been shown to reduce the risk of certain cancers, heart disease, and cataracts. They also bolster the immune system in fighting off illness. As antioxidants, these protective nutrients neutralize free radicals at the cellular level, thus protecting cell membranes, DNA, and other cellular components against damage.

The first carotenoid to be isolated was beta carotene. Today, scientists have discovered more than 600 of these protective nutrients and are reporting that many may be a hundred times more powerful than beta carotene and other antioxidants alone. The main carotenoids now under investigation are alpha carotene, cryptoxanthin, gamma carotene, lutein, and lycopene.

Alpha carotene, which makes up about one-third of the carotenoids in carrots, shows promise in inhibiting the growth of certain malignant tumors. A Japanese scientist applied alpha carotene to neuroblastoma cells (a type of childhood cancer) and observed that the nutrient began suppressing cancer growth after 18 hours. Some cells even returned to normal. In his animal studies, mice getting abundant alpha carotene developed fewer and smaller liver tumors than mice given beta carotene or no additional carotenes at all.[6]

According to ongoing research, lycopene and gamma carotene are both more powerful than vitamin E in terms of their antioxidant benefits, suggesting that they may be very protective against the tissue damage that occurs in the aftermath of exercise. Table 17-2 provides an overview of the key carotenoids, their health benefits, and food sources in which they're found.

Carotenoids

Carotenoid	Health Benefits	Food Sources
Alpha carotene	Suppresses tumor growth in certain cancers; detoxifies cancer-causing agents[7]	Carrots, pumpkin, other yellow and orange fruits and vegetables
Beta carotene	Prevents free radical damage; exerts a protective effect against cancer	Carrots, pumpkin, other yellow and orange fruits and vegetables
Gamma carotene	Exerts an antioxidant effect similar to, more powerful than vitamin E	Apricots, yellow and orange vegetables
Cryptoxanthin	Prevents damage to cell membranes and to genetic material inside cells	Oranges, tangerines, peaches, red bell peppers, yellow corn
Lutein	Essential to protect eyes from cataracts and macular degeneration (the most frequent cause of legal blindness in the U.S.)[8]	Collards, peaches, squash, kale, and turnips
Lycopene	Lowers risk of developing lung, pancreatic, bladder, and rectal cancers[9]	Tomatoes, tomato products, guava

Table 17-2

Supplementing With Carotenoids

The amount of food you consume on the Lean Bodies eating program provides a wealth of carotenoids. Foods like carrots, sweet potatoes, tomatoes, green leafy vegetables, red bell peppers, and strawberries are a treasure trove of carotenoids. But for an extra measure of protection, carotenoid supplements might be a good idea. The product I use is 3 Carotenoid Complex™, and it contains only whole food ingredients from a variety of carotenoid-rich foods.

Research has shown that the carotenoids from this particular supplement are absorbed as well as carotenoids from food. Another study with this supplement showed that it decreases lipid peroxidation in the blood that can lead to heart disease.[10]

In 1995, the USDA conducted two studies on normal, healthy people who were fed a low carotenoid diet, which included beta carotene supplements. In the first study, adding 3 Carotenoid Complex™ a day increased the immune response by 37 percent in just 20 days! This indicated that the body had a stronger ability to protect itself against harmful bacteria and viruses. In the second study, investigators measured a 20 percent increase in natural killer (NK) cells after 20 days of supplementation with 3 Carotenoid Complex™. (Part of the body's natural defense system, NK cells are a type of white blood cells that kill the sick and infectious cells in our system.[11])

Note that supplements don't replace a healthy, balanced diet. Exercising and eating whole natural foods, plus whole food supplements, are part of the Lean Bodies lifestyle. For information on 3 Carotenoid Complex™, see Appendix C.

Electrolytes

Minerals called "electrolytes" are lost through sweating during certain exercise conditions. These conditions include working out in heat and humidity, exercising for more than an hour, training at the upper levels of your VO^2 max, swimming, wearing too many clothes while working out, and taking diuretics. In any of these situations, make sure you are drinking enough water and replenishing yourself with electrolytes through your diet and supplementation.

The job of electrolytes is to regulate the body's fluid balance, both inside and outside cells. The chief electrolytes and their functions in the body are as follows:

• Sodium. Found outside cells, sodium works with potassium to keep the body's water balance in check on either side of cell walls. Both minerals are also involved in muscular contraction. Sodium can be lost if you exercise in hot weather; however, as you get used to working out in the heat, your body starts conserving sodium as a protective mechanism.

• Calcium. The most abundant mineral in the body, calcium works as an electrolyte inside cells. Calcium lost in sweat can cause muscle cramps. This mineral is best known, however, for its role in bone health and is required for the formation of bones, teeth, and other body structures. (See the following section for more information on calcium and exercise.)

• Chloride. This electrolyte acts like a lock-and-dam system by maintaining pressure to let fluids pass in and out of cells until an equilibrium is reached on both sides of the cell walls.

• Potassium. This electrolyte is found mainly inside cellular fluids. It works with sodium to help regulate the distribution of fluids on either side of cell walls. Potassium has other functions as well, including the stimulation of nerve impulses for muscular contractions, regulation of the heartbeat, the conversion of glucose to glycogen, and the synthesis of muscle protein from amino acids. Exercising in the heat can deplete potassium. But as long as you include plenty of vegetables and whole grains in your diet, potassium depletion shouldn't pose a problem.

• Magnesium. This electrolyte works inside the cellular fluid. In addition to its electrolytic function, magnesium, like other electrolytes, has many other duties in the body, including carbohydrate and protein metabolism, bone growth, and nerve function.

Of interest to people who weight train is magnesium's possible effect on strength levels. In research at Western Washington University, 26 untrained men, ages 18 to 30, participated in a study on the relationship between magnesium supplementation and strength development. Twelve subjects received a magnesium supplement; 14, a placebo. For seven weeks, they worked out three times a week, performing three sets of 10 repetitions on the leg press and leg extension. Both groups got stronger; however, there was a significant increase in strength among the supplemented group. The researchers chalked this up to magnesium's role in protein metabolism and synthesis.[12]

• Phosphorus. The second most abundant mineral in the body, phosphorus is one of the electrolytes found in the fluid inside cells. This mineral is essential for the formation of body structures, muscular contractions, nerve transmission, and kidney function. Phosphorus also plays a key role in energy production.

Supplementing With Electrolytes

Some active people rely on fluid-electrolyte sports drinks to replace lost electrolytes during exercise. A problem with many of these drinks is that they contain a lot of simple sugars such as sucrose and fructose, which are easily converted to body fat. I don't advise using these drinks because of the possible sugar overload you could experience. Instead, I use a daily mineral-electrolyte supplement to keep stores of these nutrients high. For recommended products, see Appendix A. Following the Lean Bodies eating program will also help you guard against mineral deficiencies.

Calcium

Calcium's best known role in the body is as a builder of bones and teeth. In that capacity, it has a positive effect on osteoporosis, a bone-thinning, bone-fracturing disease that strikes mostly women. On average, everyone starts losing bone around age 35, but the loss speeds up in women past menopause. This bone loss can lead to osteoporosis, but calcium — especially when combined with exercise — may help thwart it.

A number of studies confirm this, including one from Australia. Researchers there examined three treatments for osteoporosis to determine which worked the best. They selected 120 postmenopausal women and put them in an exercise group, an exercise-plus-calcium group, or an exercise-plus-estrogen group (the hormone estrogen is routinely used to treat osteoporosis). During the two-year experimental period, researchers measured the women's bone density at three forearm sites.

After all the data was compiled, it turned out that both the exercise-plus-calcium treatment and the exercise-plus-estrogen treatment slowed or prevented bone loss. The exercise-estrogen treatment was more effective, however. But the women in that group experienced unpleasant side effects, such as breast tenderness and vaginal bleeding. What this study hints at is that there is a natural way to treat bone loss — exercise and calcium supplementation — perhaps without having to resort to drugs.[13] More research is needed in this area. Talk with your physician about the latest research.

There also is a lot of data piling up that adequate calcium intake and exercise early in life help ward off bone loss later in life. A study of younger women aged 25 to 34 years old showed that a combination of regular exercise (running and walking) and high calcium intake — either by diet or supplementation — can build bone mass in the spine by up to 15 percent. The results suggest that the combination of calcium and exercise may protect against osteoporosis in later years.[14]

Supplementing With Calcium

For women, the current recommendations for calcium include maintaining a daily input of 1,000 mg before menopause and 1,500 mg daily after menopause; for men, the current recommendation is 800 mg. Younger people (ages 11 to 24) require 1,200 mg daily. Dependable sources of calcium include low-fat dairy products and green leafy vegetables. If you supplement, use an easily absorbable form of Calcium. Also Calcium needs Magnsesium in order to become soluble.

Chondroprotective Agents

If you are active, you should be concerned about protecting the health of your joints, since these structures make movement possible. One way to do that is through the use of chondroprotective agents. These are simple nutrients that help stimulate the repair of cartilage, a plastic-like tissue found throughout the body, but mainly in the joints where it works like a shock-absorber. The medical world once thought that damaged cartilage could not be repaired because it is a bloodless tissue, with no blood vessels to feed it with nutrients. But newer research shows that cartilage can heal itself, although the process is very slow. Chondroprotective agents can set this healing process in motion. The two main chondroprotective agents are glucosamine and chondroitin sulfates.

Glucosamine

Glucosamine is a type of sugar molecule manufactured naturally by cartilage cells from glucose and the amino acid, glutamine. In the presence of severe joint damage, cartilage cells may benefit from constituents such as glucosamine.

An overwhelming number of medical studies, most of them conducted in Europe, show that when dietary glucosamine is taken in supplemental form, the extra glucosamine reverses this destructive process and stimulates the cartilage cells to rebuild cartilage. Supplemental glucosamine is absorbed directly into the bloodstream, through the joint fluid and structures, eventually diffusing into the cartilage. Glucosamine has proved effective for treating osteoarthritis (a type of arthritis in which cartilage gradually deteriorates), sports injuries, and wounds. In fact, it is first-line therapy for treating osteoarthritis in several European countries.

Commercial preparations of glucosamine come in three varieties: glucosamine hydrochloride, glucosamine sulfate, and N-acetylglucosamine (NAG). Of the three, the preferred choice is glucosamine hydrochloride because it contains a higher concentration of glucosamine.

Glucosamine is not taken every day, as some supplements are. It's used to alleviate joint pain and associated problems. The recommended usage of glucosamine is 1,500 mg divided into two doses (one taken in the morning, the other at night) until your symptoms decrease. As you improve, you can cut back to 1,000 mg daily, and then to 500 mg daily. When your symptoms disappear, stop taking it all together. Ask your physician to review the research on glucosamine before you try it, and then use it in concert with standard therapies for joint problems.

Chondroitin Sulfates

Chondroitin sulfates are found naturally in cartilage and other connective tissues. Researchers discovered their effectiveness when they sprinkled cartilage powder on healing bones and skin wounds. Much to their surprise, they found that the healing process accelerated. Turns out, the active ingredient in the cartilage powder was chondroitin sulfates.[15]

As supplements, chondroitin sulfates are manufactured from cow cartilage, shark cartilage, and whale cartilage. These supplements have been shown to stimulate the production of cartilage, improve joint mobility in osteoarthritis patients, and relieve joint pain.

Research with human subjects suggests that taking one gram a day of chondroitin sulfates (divided into two doses) works best. This supplement is available in health food stores, but it's difficult to find a product that's pure.

Cosamin

The purest form of chondroitin sulfates is a product known as Cosamin™, which is actually a mixture of chondroitin sulfates and glucosamine. It contains 250 mg of chondroitin sulfates, 250 mg of glucosamine, and 50 mg of manganese, a trace mineral that activates the enzymes required to make cartilage.

Cosamin has been used with amazing success to treat joint injuries. You can get it through pharmacies or physicians, but not from health food stores since it is made from pharmaceutical-grade ingredients not available to supplement manufacturers. The usual dosage is six capsules daily.

For the best explanation of how to use chondroprotective agents and other nutrients for joint health, I suggest you read the book *Pain Free: The Definitive Guide to Healing Arthritis, Low-Back Pain, and Sports Injuries Through Nutrition and Supplements* by Luke Bucci, Ph.D. (The Summit Publishing Group, 1995).

18

Energy Optimizers

ON THE LEAN BODIES WORKOUT, you are gradually increasing your exercise intensity. Plus, you are adding another component — either aerobics or weight training — to your overall exercise program. You are also increasing the duration and frequency of your exercise sessions. In all cases, proper fueling — starting with the Lean Bodies eating program — is absolutely vital. Along with food, certain supplements can help you push harder, train longer, build muscle faster, and recover more rapidly. The following supplements may help you achieve your goal of getting leaner, faster. I personally make use of some of the following supplements:

Liquid Carbohydrate Supplements

The primary purpose of using a liquid carbohydrate supplement on the Lean Bodies Workout is to provide an extra source of energy and to help the body re-synthesize muscle glycogen. Consider a carbohydrate supplement at three critical times:

Before exercise: One sure-fire way to energize yourself for a workout is to drink a liquid carbohydrate beverage about one hour before you exercise. Studies have shown that this can maximize your performance by as much as 13 percent.[1]

During exercise: Supplementation with a liquid carbohydrate during exercise boosts your stamina by helping to maintain blood glucose, which provides fuel for the muscles and the central nervous system.

After exercise: The time you need to recover between exercise sessions often depends on how quickly your body can replenish its muscle glycogen stores. Even on the best of diets, this process can take as long as 20 hours.[2] So if you're doing aerobics twice a day to jump-start fat-burning, you could fizzle out too early to do any good.

Try to consume carbohydrates within 15 to 30 minutes of an intense workout. During this time, blood is coursing quickly through the exercised muscles, facilitating the uptake of glucose by muscle cells.

The Best Carbohydrate Formula

Although there are plenty of carbohydrate supplements on the market, your best bet is one containing maltodextrin as the sole or primary carbohydrate. Derived from starch, maltodextrin is a "slow-release" carb, meaning that it releases into the bloodstream more slowly than simple sugars like glucose and sucrose. They release into the bloodstream immediately, causing a rapid rise in blood sugar and a burst of insulin. Because of this, two things are likely to happen. First, you could experience a rapid sugar high, followed by a fast crash. This reaction will sap you of energy, and the last thing you'll feel like doing is working out.

Second, because simple sugars are released faster than the body can burn them for energy or store them as glycogen, insulin causes the excess to be converted to body fat.

As a complex carbohydrate, maltodextrin causes neither of these two reactions. Instead, it produces a more moderate insulin reaction and a more uniform energy level. Consequently, maltodextrin is not as likely to be converted to fat. On the Lean Bodies eating program, I use a carbohydrate/protein powder blend as my "mock meal," eaten at mid-morning or mid-afternoon. For a list of the carbohydrate supplements recommended on the Lean Bodies Workout, see Appendix C.

Protein Powders

Protein powders can be used as a low-fat, economical source of extra protein in your diet, especially if you need to pump up your protein intake. When I'm low in protein for the day I add some additional protein powder to my mock meal drink (see the Appendix for recommended products).

The combination of protein and carbohydrates in supplement form can give you a real advantage while following the Lean Bodies Workout. This combination appears to enhance two important energy systems of the body — the phosphagen system and the glycolytic energy system during short, powerful bursts of activity such as weight training.

If you recall, in the phosphagen system, a molecular fuel called ATP is generated. ATP, short for adenosine triphosphate, is made naturally from the nutrients in food. All cells, including muscle cells, run on ATP. This system fuels muscular activity for only a few seconds of activity at the most.

Supplementing with a carb-protein formula appears to stimulate your body's phosphagen energy system. In a study at the University of Connecticut Human Performance Laboratory, 12 active college men took a dietary supplement consisting of amino acids, ribose (a special type of sugar), and other nutrients. This supplement provided 15 grams of protein, 45 grams of carbohydrate, 5 grams of fat, and 1 gram of fiber. The subjects drank the supplement daily for 14 days straight. After the 14-day period, they had no supplement for three weeks. They then took a placebo for another 14 day period.

To check the effects of the supplement on performance, exercise tests were performed prior to and following the 14 days of supplementation and placebo ingestion. The men worked out on a cycle ergometer (a bicycle designed to measure the work performed by muscles) that could be adjusted to increase resistance.

Five minutes after each exercise test, the researchers collected blood samples to measure the concentration of ATP. Turns out that drinking the supplement for 14 days boosted pre-exercise levels of ATP in the blood. What's more, the subjects were able to work out harder after supplementation than they were after taking the placebo.[3] The point is that these participants used a supplement added to their food intake and received benefits from it. Nothing replaces food as fuel. If the participants had added the same amount of energy with food they would have seen equal or better results. However to me, this study shows how convenient supplementation can be when used with food for performance.

A carb-protein supplement has also been shown to enhance the glycolytic system. The addition of protein accelerates your body's glycogen-making machinery. In fact, when you take protein with carbs as a post-workout supplement, more glycogen is taken up and stored by your muscles. That means you can store more carbohydrate energy. With more glycogen around, you have a ready source of fuel for muscular contractions. Conversely, fatigue sets in when you're low on glycogen.

The message in all of this? Try mixing your carbohydrate supplement with your protein powder for an energy-enhancing boost. For recommendations on supplemental protein powders, see Appendix C.

Sports Nutrition Bars

Sports nutrition bars are fast becoming the most popular supplement for exercisers and athletes today. Available at gyms, health food stores, and grocery stores, these candy bar-like products are specially formulated with protein, carbohydrates, fats, and other nutrients — all to provide a nutritional and performance boost for exercise.

The sports nutrition bar market is expanding so rapidly that it's often difficult to know which product is the best for your needs. Many bars are as high in fat and simple sugars as a standard candy bar — definitely not what you need when trying to get lean and firm. As for calories, the range is wide. Some bars have as few as 130 calories; others go as high as 500 calories. Among major nutrients, the carbohydrate content ranges from 100 grams to 16 grams; protein, from 30 grams down to 1 gram. As for fat, the content varies from as high as 7 grams per bar to 1 gram per bar. Some bars are vitamin-fortified.

So what's the best bar for you, especially on the Lean Bodies Workout? The bar we use at Lean Bodies is the Parrillo Supplement Bar. A survey conducted on the nutritional content of 27 bars on the market helped me substantiate the use of this bar on our program. Of the bars surveyed, 25 contained fructose, corn syrup, concentrated fruit juice, or other simple sugar as the main ingredient. Thirteen of the bars were high in fat. Here's the problem: Concentrated fructose, simple sugars, and fats are the least optimal foods to include in a proper diet. In the body, they convert easily to body fat because of the way they're metabolized if you have a slower metabolism.

We're not alone in our opinion, either. Not long ago, the *Cincinnati Enquirer* did a story on sports nutrition bars and rated the Parrillo Supplement Bar the best for taste. That's a plus, especially since most bars we've tried have an unpleasant "vitamin" taste.

I'm personally convinced of its nutritional merit because the bar is formulated scientifically with ingredients that make it unique on the market. Each 240-calorie bar provides 38 grams of complex carbohydrate from the glucose polymer rice dextrin, a complex carbohydrate that releases into the bloodstream at just the right rate to maintain a uniform energy level. Also, the bar contains only one gram of conventional fat.

The Parrillo Supplement Bar also contains 11 grams of two high quality proteins, casein and lactalbumin. Working together with carbs, protein helps speed up the body's glycogen-making process, as well as maintain blood sugar so you don't have energy-sapping, low-blood sugar dips during the day.

Another ingredient that sets this product apart is that it contains 5.5 grams of pure MCT oil, a special type of dietary fat that is used immediately for energy and is not stored as body fat (see Chapter 20). Along with its complex carbs, the MCT oil makes this sports nutrition bar a highly concentrated source of fuel. The chocolate version of the bar is flavored with naturally sweet, defatted cocoa. Other flavors include vanilla, peanut butter, and layered chocolate peanut butter.

Convenient to pack in a gym bag or purse, the bar can be eaten with meals as an additional source of calories, between meals as a delicious and nutritious snack, or after workouts to supply the nutrients required for recovery. Plus, this product is an excellent way to gradually increase your calories for a metabolic boost. On the Lean Bodies eating program, our clients have had great results when they make the bar their mock meal between breakfast and lunch, or between lunch and dinner. Be sure to drink plenty of water with the bar, too, since fluid helps speed the bar's nutrients from your digestive tract into your bloodstream.

Creatine

Discovered in 1832, creatine is a constituent of muscles, where it plays a role in the transfer of energy in muscle cells and in the production of ATP for muscular contractions. Inside the muscles, it is converted into creatine phosphate (CP), a small energy supply for muscles. CP also regenerates ATP.

More than 95 percent of the creatine in your body is stored in your muscles. Your body can synthesize creatine from the amino acids, arginine, glycine, and methionine. On average, a 154-pound man naturally uses up about 2 grams of creatine a day, an amount that can be easily replaced by food, specifically fish and meat. [4]

Creatine levels in the muscle can be increased with supplementation, and this enhances the phosphagen energy system. Studies have shown that creatine-loading in this manner improves performance in short-burst, high-intensity activities such as weight training and sprinting, in which CP typically supplies energy. But creatine doesn't work as well in endurance sports, where the body relies more on muscle glycogen and fat for fuel.

Exercisers who supplement with creatine can work out harder, longer, and with greater strength. It appears to reduce muscle soreness as well, by zapping free radicals caused by exercise. There's less tissue damage as a result — and less muscle soreness. Some exercisers and athletes report that creatine causes water retention.

As a supplement, creatine comes in the form of creatine monohydrate. You take it by dissolving one teaspoon (about 5 grams) in water two to three times a day and drinking this solution to super-saturate your muscles. If you choose, supplement in this manner during periods when you are weight training on a regular basis. Remember, food is first and foremost.

Branched-Chain Amino Acids

The "branched-chain amino acids," or BCAAs for short, are leucine, valine, and isoleucine. Their chief role is to assist the muscles in synthesizing other amino acids for growth and repair.

They are also used to provide energy, but only under special circumstances. If you do high-intensity aerobics for an hour or longer, the BCAAs, particularly leucine, get involved in energy production. In a series of events, leucine is broken down to make another amino acid, alanine. Alanine is then turned into glucose to supply energy to your exercising muscles.

BCAAs are becoming increasingly important as supplemental nutrients for exercisers, especially since research shows that these amino acids can improve performance. Supplemental BCAAs taken before and during exercise have been shown to prevent excessive breakdown of muscle protein.[5,6] What that means to you is this: With more BCAAs supplied to the body, there's less protein lost from muscles. Ultimately, that means your body can repair itself better following exercise.

BCAAs also appear to affect the response of certain muscle-building hormones during exercise. A case in point: 14 long-distance runners, ages 24 to 42, participated in two different experiments, conducted a week apart. In the first experiment, the runners were given a BCAA supplement just prior to one hour of continuous running. In the second experiment, they received a placebo.

By taking a series of blood samples before, during, and after the experiments, the researchers found that several hormones, including growth hormone, were elevated in all the runners — in both experiments. The most notable difference concerned testosterone levels. Testosterone is a sex hormone responsible for the development of male characteristics, including muscular development. Without BCAA supplementation, testosterone levels declined. But with supplementation, it increased during the recovery period. These findings led the researchers to conclude that BCAA supplementation before exercise affects the response of testosterone and other tissue-building hormones.[7]

Clearly, BCAAs show promise as supplemental nutrition for exercisers and athletes. If you supplement with BCAAs, don't take them on an empty stomach. Branched-chain aminos require insulin from the release of carbohydrates in order to move into the muscles, and, therefore, must be taken with meals.

Coenzyme Q$_{10}$ — An Antioxidant
For Improving Aerobic Performance

This dietary supplement, a compound which the body also synthesizes on its own, is widely prescribed in Japan as an adjunct to medication for heart disease. Among other functions, coenzyme Q$_{10}$ (abbreviated as CoQ$_{10}$) is an antioxidant that helps improve cardiac function, lower cholesterol, and strengthen the immune system.

Coenzyme Q$_{10}$ is a compound directly involved in energy-producing reactions that ultimately generate ATP, the molecular fuel for cells. It resides in the mitochondria and membranes of cells.

Well-scrutinized in many scientific studies, CoQ$_{10}$ may be a major energy booster for exercisers and athletes, since it can saturate muscle tissue, a condition that improves aerobic power. Indeed, some of CoQ$_{10}$'s clinical reports sound truly remarkable:

• Nine middle-aged women who tired easily took CoQ$_{10}$ supplements (90 mg daily) for six months. None of the women was anemic nor had any cardiovascular problems, two medical causes of fatigue. During the study period, the women were tested on treadmills to see how long they could go before becoming exhausted. At the three-month and six-month points in the study, the women increased their exercise time before fatiguing. Plus, their VO$_2$ max improved significantly. Five of the nine women had fewer symptoms of fatigue, and three women became normal, thanks to supplementation with CoQ$_{10}$.[8]

• Ten sedentary people and nine aerobically fit volleyball players took 100 mg a day of CoQ$_{10}$ for 30 days, followed by three weeks without it. All the subjects were tested on a cycle ergometer to check the effects of supplementation. After the supplementation period, significant increases in work capacity, VO$_2$ max, and plasma levels of CoQ$_{10}$ were detected in all the subjects. The findings show that CoQ$_{10}$ works well as an aerobic booster for both sedentary and active people.[9]

• Ten male professional basketball players were put into two groups of five each. One group served as a control; the other took CoQ$_{10}$ supplements (100 mg daily) for 40 days. All the players trained as usual. After the study, researchers measured the players' VO$_2$ max, plus heart function. VO$_2$ max increased significantly (18 percent) among the supplemented players, but not in the control group. Also, cardiac efficiency, as well as the pumping action of the heart, was greatly improved in the supplemented athletes.[10]

These are just a few of the many studies on CoQ$_{10}$ showing that this supplement does indeed supercharge athletic activity and may be worth adding to your nutrition program to push your performance up a notch or more.

Supplementing With CoQ$_{10}$

Thanks to thorough documentation in thousands of subjects, supplemental CoQ$_{10}$ appears to be safe for long-term use. You can purchase the supplement from health food stores, mail order supplement companies, and sporting goods stores. The usual recommended dosage is 60 to 200 mg a day. Before considering the use of supplemental CoQ$_{10}$, consult your physician.

19

Lipotropics For Mobilizing Fat

TECHNICALLY, "lipotropic" refers to any substance that decreases the rate at which fat is stored in liver cells and accelerates the rate at which fat is dismantled into water, carbon dioxide, and energy. The nutrients described below are all important lipotropics, with known fat-mobilizing abilities. Used in conjunction with the Lean Bodies program and Lean Bodies Workout, they can help prevent fat from accumulating faster than your body can use it. By helping to mobilize fat, lipotropics make fat fully available for energy, thus assisting in fat loss.

Choline

Present in all living cells, choline is considered a member of the vitamin B-complex family. In the body, choline is synthesized from the interaction of two B-complex vitamins, vitamin B_{12} and folic acid, with the amino acid methionine. It works together with another lipotropic, inositol, to prevent fat from building up in the liver and to move fat into cells to be burned for energy.

Choline also plays a role in helping your body better utilize cholesterol. Within the liver, choline is involved in the formation of lecithin, a natural constituent of cells that helps emulsify cholesterol.

Choline is important to the health of the myelin sheaths of the nerves. These sheaths insulate and protect nerve fibers, which are responsible for transmitting messages. If the myelin sheath is damaged, nerve fibers can't heal or regenerate themselves and will stop functioning.

Many animal and plant proteins contain hefty amounts of choline, so insufficient protein in the diet can cause a deficiency. This can lead to a range of health problems, including fatty deposits in the liver, cirrhosis of the liver, kidney problems, high blood pressure, and hardening of the arteries.

Inositol

Like choline, inositol is a B-complex vitamin. It's involved primarily in promoting the production of lecithin in the body so that fat metabolism can proceed normally. Working together with choline, inositol helps prevent dangerous accumulations of fat in the arteries and keeps the liver, heart, and kidneys healthy.

You also need inositol for normal functioning of body cells. This nutrient is required by cells in the bone marrow, eye membranes, and intestines for proper growth.

Your body can make inositol from glucose (blood sugar), and the nutrient is plentiful in whole grains. Too much coffee can deplete your body's reservoir of inositol. Deficiencies of inositol can cause eczema, constipation, and eye problems.

Carnitine

Carnitine is a protein-like nutrient that shuttles fat into the mitochondria of cells to be burned for energy. Produced in the liver and kidneys, carnitine is made from lysine and methionine, two amino acids, through a series of interactions with vitamin C, vitamin B_3, and vitamin B_6.

Of interest is the fact that carnitine is found in foods that are also high in fat, namely red meat. Scientists believe it exists there for a good purpose — to help the person who eats meat better break down the fat in meat. Fish has a little carnitine, and the fattier portions of chicken such as the leg have more carnitine than the breast. Several vegetable foods contain carnitine, and these include wheat germ and cauliflower. Carnitine is quite vulnerable to heat and is easily destroyed by cooking.

About one-fifth of your carnitine requirements can be met by eating red meat. But since most commercial red meat is high in fat, supplementation may be helpful.

Carnitine For Exercise Performance

Carnitine has been found to boost exercise performance by making more fat available to working muscles. Researchers in Romania gave carnitine to 110 top athletes (rowers, kayakers, swimmers, weight lifters, and long distance runners) and found the supplementation caused more fatty acids to enter cells to be used as energy. With a larger amount of fat available for energy, conceivably performance can be improved. Based on their findings, the researchers recommended carnitine supplementation as an ergogenic (performance-enhancing) aid, especially for endurance and strength sports.[2]

Another Romanian study looked into the effects of carnitine supplementation on competitive junior cyclists. Seven top cyclists were given 2 grams of carnitine daily 10 days prior to competition, along with extra protein (1 gram per kg of bodyweight) for six weeks; seven other cyclists received a placebo. Favorable changes were observed in the supplemented group:

Strength went up, lean mass increased, and body fat was scaled back. What's more, the supplemented group performed better than the placebo group in the international competition that took place at the end of the experiment. For competitive athletes, the researchers recommend increasing protein intake (up to 3.2 grams per kg) six weeks before competition and supplementing with 2 grams of carnitine daily beginning 10 to 14 days before competing, including the day of competition. Carnitine, they believe, improves the "biological potential" of the body.[3]

Other scientists believe that carnitine enhances exercise performance in other ways, besides mobilizing of fat. Evidence is surfacing that carnitine increases VO_2 max (aerobic capacity) and reduces the buildup of waste products like lactic acid in the muscles, thereby extending performance.

Carnitine And Immunity

Carnitine may also affect immune response. One study shows that carnitine increased the response of lymphocytes, an infection-fighting white blood cell formed in the body's lymphatic system, and neutralized the lipid-induced immunosuppression.[4]

Carnitine And Heart Health

Carnitine may play a critical role in cardiovascular health, too. The heart prefers to burn fat for fuel, unlike muscles, which can run on either fat or carbohydrate. In the heart, carnitine acts like a fuel injection system, supplying heart cells with fat for fuel. When the heart muscle is damaged in some way, its carnitine supply is depleted. In heart patients, studies have shown that carnitine helps protect against heart rhythm irregularities, could reduce angina attacks, could lower blood fats, and could increase HDL cholesterol (the good kind).[5]

Safety Issues

The L-carnitine form of this supplement appears to be safe. However, another form, D-carnitine, is not safe. D-carnitine also causes depletion of L-carnitine.[6] Some supplement preparations contain combinations of the L and D forms, so be careful. If you supplement with carnitine, use products that contain L-carnitine only.

Chromium

Even though your body requires chromium in only the tiniest amounts (50 to 200 mcg daily), this trace nutrient is essential for normal sugar and fat metabolism. It has the ability to help the hormone insulin do a better job of transporting glucose (blood sugar) and amino acids across cell membranes.

By assisting insulin in amino acid uptake, chromium has an indirect effect on muscle growth. And like many minerals, chromium activates enzymes involved in protein synthesis.

Chromium also helps regulate the synthesis of fat. When excess insulin is released, your body can go into a fat-producing mode. Insulin secretion triggers the activity of lipoprotein lipase, the enzyme that tells fat cells to start making fat. By making insulin work better, chromium, in effect, inhibits fat synthesis.

Certain factors can cause both marginal and serious deficiencies of chromium, and these include high-sugar diets and strenuous exercise.[7] The proof of this is in studies in which scientists have measured chromium losses in the urine of exercisers on training days. They have found that urinary losses are the highest on those days.[8] If you don't get enough chromium — and you're working out consistently and vigorously — then you're risking your chromium status.

High-sugar diets compromise chromium status, too. In one study, 37 people (19 men and 18 women) were fed healthy diets with optimal levels of protein, carbohydrates, fat, and other nutrients for 12 weeks. Afterward, for six weeks, the subjects were put on a high-sugar diet (15 percent of the total calories were from simple sugars). In 27 of the 37 subjects, urinary chromium losses increased 30-fold. The lesson here is that too much sugar in the diet can lead to a chromium deficiency, possibly interfering with your body's ability to use glucose properly and burn fat.[9]

Chromium used to be plentiful in certain foods, namely whole grain cereals and vegetables. But modern farming methods have stripped the soil of nutrients, including chromium, so that it's difficult to get enough of this mineral from processed/refined foods. Note, Brewer's Yeast is a good source of chromium.

Biotin

Biotin is a B-complex vitamin involved in the metabolism of fats. Without it, the body can't properly burn fats. Although required in tiny amounts (150 to 300 mcg daily), biotin can be in short supply — for two reasons. First, the best sources of biotin in food are egg yolks and liver — two foods we tend to cut back on because of their high concentration of cholesterol. Second, research verifies that active people often have lower levels of biotin than others. A possible reason has to do with exercise. Exercising causes the waste product lactic acid to accumulate in working muscles. Biotin is involved in the process that breaks down lactic acid. The more lactic acid that builds up in muscles, the more biotin that is needed to break it down.[10]

A dietary practice that interferes with the body's use of biotin is eating raw eggs (which also puts you at risk of contracting salmonella poisoning). Raw egg whites contain a protein called avidin that binds with biotin and keeps it from being absorbed. Cooking eggs inactivates avidin.

Supplementing with biotin — either through a multi-vitamin formula or lipotropic supplement — offers an extra measure of protection against a possible deficiency.

Other Lipotropic Agents

Because of the role they play in fat metabolism, chromium (in the form of chromium picolinate), carnitine, inositol, choline, and biotin are the most common lipotropics found in supplemental preparations. Two other lipotropics found in supplements include betaine, a substance from which choline is formed; and methionine, an amino acid that, like choline, helps mobilize fat.

Supplementing With Lipotropics

If you decide to supplement with a lipotropic supplement as part of the Lean Bodies Workout, choose a product that contains at least the "big five" — chromium, carnitine, inositol, choline, and biotin. (See Appendix C for product recommendations.) Depending on the manufacturer's suggestion for usage, lipotropic supplements are usually taken with meals.

20

Special Lipids For Exercisers

YOU WOULDN'T THINK that a "lipid," otherwise known as a fat, would be beneficial in an exercise program geared for fat loss. True, you want to keep your dietary fat intake low (around 10 percent of your total daily calories or less) to shed body fat. However, there are two types of dietary fats that can enhance your results and performance on the Lean Bodies Workout if used correctly. These fats are omega-3 fatty acids and MCT oil.

Omega-3 Fatty Acids

For more than 20 years, research reports have been pouring in over the potent health benefits of fish oils, namely omega-3 fatty acids found primarily in deep-sea fish. There are non-fish sources, too, and these include flaxseed oil, canola oil, and soybean oil. The two most beneficial members of the omega-3 family are eicosapentanoic acid (EPA) and docosa-hexanoic acid (DHA).

Their healthful properties first came to light when scientists discovered that Eskimos have a lower rate of heart disease and stroke than other populations, despite their high-fat diet. The difference is that Eskimos eat 20 times more fish than most Americans do, and fish is full of omega-3 fatty acids.

Because of this link, omega-3 fatty acids have become best known for their good deeds in cardiovascular health, where they have been found to lower blood pressure, reduce cholesterol, thwart dangerous blood clotting, and protect against irregular heartbeats.

Omega-3 fatty acids are important in joint health as well, because they're required for the production of prostaglandins. Prostaglandins are hormone-like biochemicals derived from the essential fatty acid, arachidonic acid. They assist the immune system in preventing infection, reducing inflammation, and fighting disease. Studies have shown that fish oils may be particularly effective in cases of rheumatoid arthritis, a crippling form of arthritis in which the body's own immune system attacks itself.

There can occur not-so-friendly prostaglandins in the body, too, which may be involved in osteoarthritis and cancerous tissue growth. The body's cells make this particular type of prostaglandin from saturated fats. But in a rather dramatic nutritional rescue, omega-3 fatty acids interfere with their manufacture by grabbing on to an enzyme that harmful prostaglandins need for production. The more of the enzyme these fish oils can take, the less there is to make these nasty prostaglandins.

Omega-3 fatty acids are richest in mackerel, salmon, trout, tuna, and sardines. One type of fish oil — salmon oil — dramatically reduces triglycerides, cholesterol, and a harmful type of cholesterol known as VLDL (very-low-density lipoproteins) in people with an excess of blood fats in their system. Salmon oil has also been shown to increase HDL cholesterol, the beneficial kind.[1]

Omega-3 Fatty Acids And Exercise Performance

In addition to heart and joint health, omega-3 fatty acids have been studied for their role in exercise performance. In 1988, an entire college football team started supplementing with an omega-3 fatty acid supplement eight times a day, with record-smashing results. On average, the team's bench press repetitions increased 10.2 percent; number of chin-ups, 9.3 percent; and vertical jumps, up 2.6 percent. They were able to shave their 300-yard shuttle times by 3 percent and make improvements in their heart rates. Clearly, supplementation improved strength and aerobic performance. Similar results with other football teams led to the endorsement of a particular omega-3 fatty acid supplement by the NFL Players Association as a nutritional alternative to anabolic (tissue-building) drugs.[2]

Football players are one type of athlete, but what about the rest of us — people who work out mainly for fitness? A university study sheds some light on this. In a study of 32 healthy men, researchers found that supplementation with omega-3 fatty acids mimics the effects of aerobic exercise.[3]

Also, omega-3 fatty acids have the ability to dilate the capillaries. This improves the flow of oxygen and nutrients to muscles during exercise, as well as capillary vasodilation.[4] The more nutrients the muscles can get, the better the conditions are for growth and repair.

Because of their role in the production of good prostaglandins, omega-3 fatty acids may also reduce exercise-caused inflammation and allow you to recover faster following exercise.

Supplementing With Omega-3 Fatty Acids

By far one of the best omega-3 supplements is salmon oil. It is the richest, purest source of these important fatty acids you can find. The product I use is Neo-Life Salmon Oil. Suggested usage can be found on the bottle.

Beneficial Effects Of Omega-3 Fatty Acids On
Exercise Performance

- Joint health protection.
- Alleviation of exercise-caused inflammation and improved recovery.
- Enhanced delivery of oxygen and nutrients to muscles, efficient removal of waste products.
- Increased VO_2 max.

Table 20-1

MCT Oil

MCT (medium chain triglyceride) oil is a specially engineered dietary oil discussed at length in the first Lean Bodies book and used in my eating program.

Thanks to its unique molecular structure, MCT oil is burned immediately for energy and therefore has little tendency to be able to be stored as body fat as conventional fats and oils are. MCT oil is rapidly processed into energy that is lost as body heat in a process called thermogenesis, which elevates the metabolism. When calories are given off as body heat, fewer are left to be packed away as fat.

MCT oil can do something else regular fats can't: enter the mitochondria of cells when carbohydrate is present. In the presence of carbohydrates, MCTs are burned for energy — another reason why they aren't easily stored as body fat. Also, the burning of MCTs in the mitochondria makes more carbohydrates available for energy, thus increasing endurance and stamina.

You can use MCT oil as a source of extra calories (114 per tablespoon) so that you can train longer and harder — and develop body-toning muscle as a result. Lean Bodies participants who take MCT oil love it, because of the energy it gives them.

MCT oil can be used on my Two-Week Fat-Burning Blitz. On this plan, you exclude starchy carbohydrates in the evening — a measure that suppresses the release of insulin but kicks in glucagon, which unlocks fat stores for energy. Sometimes, excluding carbs at night can cause a dip in energy levels. Compensate by using MCT oil, taken with food in the afternoon, with mini-meals, or in the evening.

How To Take MCT Oil

MCT oil should always be taken with food and can be poured over vegetables. You can also cook or bake with MCT oil just as you would with any other vegetable oil. Keep the heat at 350 degrees or lower, however, because MCT oil smokes at high temperatures. Don't store MCT oil in anything other than a glass container. It tends to soften containers made of certain types of plastic.

Gradually introduce MCT oil into your diet at the rate of a few teaspoons a day. This supplement is so rapidly absorbed that it tends to cause stomach cramping if too much is taken at one time or on an empty stomach.

Make sure you purchase pure MCT oil, not a product that's diluted. How can you tell? A good rule of thumb is that any MCT oil product that comes flavored is not the pure stuff. Also, simply read the label to see whether the product is cut with flavorings or other fillers. At Lean Bodies, we've found that anyone who has used a flavored MCT oil simply doesn't get the same results.

As with any supplement, you should consult your physician before taking MCT oil. This is especially true for diabetics or individuals with a condition called ketosis.

Beneficial Effects Of MCT Oil On Exercise Performance

• Immediately available source of energy.

• Little tendency to be stored as body fat, unlike conventional fats and oil.

• Affects metabolic rate through thermogenesis.

• Ability to spare carbohydrates.

• Fat-burning.

Table 20-2

21

Desiccated Liver: Nutrient Treasure Trove For Lean Bodies Exercisers

ONE OF THE BEST ALL-AROUND supplements for active people is desiccated liver, a concentrated form of beef liver that has been processed to remove the cholesterol but to preserve the nutrient content of the liver. It comes in tablet form, and the more advanced products are fortified with other nutrients. Desiccated liver is an important supplemental source of iron, a critical mineral for exercisers and athletes. It is also naturally rich in B-complex vitamins; vitamins A, B, C, and D; calcium; and phosphorus, with four times the nutritional value in the same amount of cooked whole liver.

In animal studies, desiccated liver has been shown to enhance endurance and increase strength. In one study, three groups of rats were fed controlled diets for three months. One group consumed a basic diet supplemented with vitamins and minerals; the second group ate the same diet, along with B-complex vitamins and brewer's yeast; and the third group ate the basic diet, supplemented with desiccated liver. The rats were placed in water to see how long they could swim before drowning. Group 1 swam an average of 13.2 minutes; and group 2, an average of 13.4 minutes. Remarkably, the desiccated liver-supplemented were still swimming at the end of two hours — ten times longer than the other two groups.[1]

Let's take a closer look at the key nutritional components of desiccated liver and why they're so essential for active people.

Iron

The major job of iron in the body is to combine with protein and copper (a trace mineral) to manufacture hemoglobin, a component of red blood cells that carries oxygen in the blood from the lungs to the tissues. Without enough hemoglobin, tissues are deprived of oxygen, often resulting in fatigue, breathlessness, and a rapid heartbeat.

Iron is also required for the formation of myoglobin, which is located in muscle tissue only. Myoglobin supplies oxygen to muscle cells so that the necessary chemical reactions can take place to make your muscles contract.

There are two types of iron. One is "heme iron," found only in liver and lean red meat, oysters, poultry, and fish. Of these, liver is really the best source. Liver is an excellent food, but only very active people with fast metabolisms can handle it, since it's high in fat and cholesterol. Desiccated liver supplements give you all the nutrition of iron, but without the fat and cholesterol. Heme iron is the easiest iron for your body to absorb.

The other kind of iron is "non-heme iron," and it's found primarily in green leafy vegetables and whole grains. There's some non-heme iron in meats, too. Non-heme iron is not as well-absorbed as heme iron is. Normally, only about 5 percent of non-heme iron in foods is absorbed, compared to about 25 percent for heme iron. One way to improve the absorption of non-heme iron is by eating vitamin C-rich foods with it. Vitamin C can more than double the amount of non-heme iron absorbed.

Exercise And Iron Status

It's imperative for good health and performance that you get ample iron in your diet, especially since exercise can partially deplete iron stores. In Spain, researchers studied a group of cadets who underwent intensive military drills for seven days to see what effect this level of physical exertion had on their iron stores. They found that iron stores were depleted, although not to the point of hindering the production of red blood cells.[2]

In another study, researchers tested 12 healthy college men who exercised on a stationary bicycle as part of the experiment. Blood samples were drawn at rest and at the end of the exercise bout and measured for various indications of iron depletion. What decreased significantly after exercise were the subjects' iron stores.[3]

If you're not well-nourished, weight training can affect iron status, too, especially when you first start. A study of 12 unexercised men who started a weight training program showed an initial depletion of iron stores after six weeks of training for two hours a day, four times a week.[4]

Eating foods rich in iron, such as lean red meats, dark leafy greens, and possibly dessicated liver, may be of benefit to the strenuous exerciser.

Iron Deficiency Issues

Active women are especially vulnerable to iron deficiencies. One reason is that women don't get enough iron in their diets. The recommended dietary allowance (RDA) for iron is 15 mg daily for women. On average, American diets contain 5 to 7 mg of iron per 1,000 calories.

An iron deficiency can lead to full-fledged anemia, which literally means "no blood." If you are anemic, your hemoglobin levels are below normal, and your blood lacks enough oxygen-carrying red blood cells. Every tissue and organ in your body is literally starved for oxygen.

As you might imagine, anemia harms physical performance — in several ways. It reduces VO_2 max, lowers endurance, and increases the buildup of energy-sapping waste products in the muscle. These conditions can all spell fatigue. If you think you have full-fledged anemia, a blood test can confirm or deny it.

You may have heard of "sports anemia," a condition characterized by a drop in hemoglobin levels. It has been observed in elite endurance athletes, couch potatoes who start exercising, and exercisers who increase their exercise intensity. Exactly how sports anemia occurs is unclear, although there are two suspected causes.

First, during the early phases of an aerobic exercise program or a competitive endurance training regimen, the body adapts to the exercise by using more protein to make myoglobin and other protein compounds the muscles need to properly use oxygen. If protein is in short supply, the body starts destroying red blood cells to synthesize myoglobin. There's a resulting decline in hemoglobin. Consuming adequate protein (20 to 25 percent of total daily calories) can prevent this from happening.

The second explanation for sports anemia has to do with blood volume, the amount of blood in your body. Exercise helps promote a slight increase in blood volume, diluting — but not changing — the amount of hemoglobin in the blood. You can look at it this way: While sipping a glass of iced tea, you find it tastes too strong, so you add some water. You change the liquid volume in your glass, but you don't change the amount of actual tea. It works the same way with blood volume and hemoglobin. In a blood test, hemoglobin appears to be in low concentrations, when in fact, it's not. Actually, increased blood volume is a plus, since it indicates better oxygen delivery to cells during exercise, provided enough iron is available.

There is another type of anemia that can affect exercisers — "exercise-induced hemolytic anemia." That's a mouthful, but all it means is red blood cell destruction caused by the trauma of repetitive foot strikes against hard surfaces, muscular contraction, acid conditions in the muscle, and increased body temperature. Detectable by a blood test, this form of anemia is seen mostly in middle-aged distance runners who are overweight, wear poorly cushioned shoes, and run hard on their feet. It's rarely observed in athletes who stay lean, wear proper shoes, and use good running form.[6]

Stay Iron-Healthy

Getting the iron you need from proper nutrition is clearly important to your exercise program and overall health. You can do this by eating lean red meat, particularly longhorn beef, and other low-fat cuts of meat. With your iron stores full, you can potentially increase your aerobic capacity (combined with aerobic training), extend your energy, and improve your body's recuperative powers. This all adds up to maximum performance.

Note: For information about Longhorn Beef call 1-800-697-LEAN

B-Complex Vitamins

As noted earlier, desiccated liver is a rich source of the B-complex vitamins. This family of vitamins is responsible for providing the body with energy, mainly by converting carbohydrates into glucose, an important fuel for cells. The B-complex vitamins are also essential for the metabolism of protein and fat, healthy functioning of the nervous system, maintenance of muscle tone in the gastrointestinal tract, and the health of skin, hair, eyes, mouth, and liver.

B-complex vitamins are water-soluble and therefore not stored by the body. They have to be continually replaced by diet, supplementation, or both. Some B vitamins can be lost through sweat. Coffee can cause the body to use up B vitamins, as can infection or stress. Too much sugar in the diet can destroy B vitamins.

Listed in Table 21-1 on the next page are performance-related functions of B-complex vitamins. If supplementing with B-complex vitamins, always take them together, since doses of single B vitamins can cause imbalances.

Performance-Related Functions Of The Major B-Complex Vitamins

Vitamin	Function	Best Sources	*General Usage Guidelines
B$_1$ (thiamine)	Breakdown of carbs into glucose for energy improvement of muscle tone of the heart	Desiccated liver and whole grains	.5 mg per 1000 calories daily
B$_2$ (riboflavin)	Breakdown of carbohydrates, fats, and protein; utilization of oxygen inside cells	Desiccated liver, brewer's yeast	1.6 mg (men); 1.2 mg (women)
B$_6$ (pyridoxine)	Breakdown of carbohydrates, fats, and protein; production of red blood cells; release of glycogen from liver and muscles for energy; healthy function of the musculoskeletal system	Meats, whole grains, desiccated liver, brewer's yeast	2 mg per 100 grams of protein daily
B$_{12}$	Carbohydrate, fat, and protein metabolism	Found only in animal foods	3 mcg daily

continued on page 281

Vitamin	Function	Best Sources	*General Usage Guidelines
	assistance in the healthy functioning of iron in the body; assistance in the synthesis of choline, a lipotropic (fat-burning) agent		
Folic Acid	Breakdown of protein; formation of red blood cells; growth and reproduction of cells; believed to have a preventive role in heart disease and stroke	Green leafy vegetables, desiccated liver, brewer's yeast	400 mcg.
Niacin	Breakdown of carbohydrates, fats, and protein; reduction of cholesterol; improvement of circulation	Desiccated liver, wheat germ, brewer's yeast	6.6 mg per 1000 calories daily
Pantothenic Acid	Release of energy from carbohydrates, fat, and proteins; utilization of other vitamins	Desiccated liver, whole grain cereals, brewer's yeast	5 to 10 mg daily

Table 21-1

* Check with your physician for recommended dosages of nutrients.

Part V

Making The Lean Bodies Workout Your Lifestyle

22

Team Lean: A Revolutionary New Motivational Concept

STOP AND REFLECT FOR A MOMENT. What are all the positive changes taking place now that you are getting more active and changing your eating habits? List as many as you can. For example:

• A more defined body, with less body fat.
• More lean mass.
• More energy and greater stamina.
• Improved health.
• More confident self-image.
• Better outlook on life.
• Improved sleeping patterns.

By themselves, changes like these should be self-motivating — providing enough of an inner drive to make you stick to it. If you work out for any length of time, you start to view yourself differently. You look better, feel better, perform better. Those things build and bolster confidence, and that's hard to give up.

Let's look at a Lean Body who is motivated by her super-lean figure:

"I can stay motivated by just looking in the mirror and getting all the compliments I get," says Patty E. "Also, during the summer, a friend and I work out together, then we reward ourselves by spending the rest of the day at the lake in the sun ... in bikinis!"

Exercise Motivation

But results don't always spell motivational success. About half the people who start an exercise program will drop out within the first six months, despite all the benefits.[1]

Experts agree that if you can stay with it for three weeks, then your fitness attempts will no longer be a trial. Poor commitment isn't limited to new exercisers, however. Even among veteran exercisers, willpower can flag for many reasons, including lack of time, inconvenience, cost, boredom, injuries, to name just a few.

Introducing Team Lean

At Lean Bodies, we've recognized how critical it is to rein-force exercise and proper nutrition as a lifestyle. That's why we've developed an innovative, surefire motivational system known as "Team Lean." It builds on the principle of group sup-port, a proven motivator not only in exercise but also in other fields of endeavor. Group support is a very potent part of any fitness effort.

By exercising with a group, you associate with those who enjoy exercise and can give you the companionship and positive reinforcement you need. If you're like a lot of people, exercising alone is a struggle, and you're likely to throw in the towel before you even get started.

In our Lean Bodies classes, I've found that the most consistent exercisers are the ones who work out with a partner. Often, another person's willpower may be just what you need when you're tempted to skip a workout.

Group support definitely helps you maintain the exercise habit — a fact that's been well documented by research. Studies show that people who exercise in a group are more likely to adhere to their program than those who exercise on their own. A few other cases in point:

• For six months, home exercisers who received periodic telephone calls from a research staff member boosted their aerobic capacity significantly — meaning that they stuck to the program well enough to derive physical benefits — compared to a control group which had no staff support.[2]

• Thirty-eight women were divided into two aerobic dance groups: one group received individual and group reinforcement; the other group received neither. You would expect that the reinforcement group would do better at sticking to the program, but that's not what happened. In both groups, 94 percent of the participants stayed with it.

At the end of the study, the researchers interviewed everyone to see why adherence was so high. Here are some of the reasons the women gave: The makeup of the group was similar, so the women felt comfortable with one another; they enjoyed the socializing; they were able to set goals and commit to achieving them; and they felt buoyed by their increased energy and fitness.[3]

• In a study where group competition, monitoring, and support were promoted, there was a dropout rate of only 9 percent and an adherence rate of 98 percent — one of the highest ever documented.[4]

What these and other studies confirm is that group support can provide just the extra incentive you need to persevere in your exercise program, plus get all the fitness rewards it promises.

How To Establish Your Own Team Lean

The first step in building your team is to find two, three, or four partners with whom you are compatible. They can be your friends, neighbors, business associates, or family members, and should be selected based on the following criteria:

• All of you should be "like-minded," that is, be interested in exercise, nutrition, and good health — and the benefits they bring.

• Your partners should all have similar exercise skill levels in terms of strength, endurance, and aerobic capacity.

• You should share the same workout and nutrition philosophies. It's important that you all be on the Lean Bodies eating program, so that there's no shortage of physical energy among partners and so that ideas can be shared as to recipes and personal nutrition tips.

• Each person on the team should be a "positive motivator," and not a "cheap complimentor." In other words, don't tell your partner he's looking great, when in fact he has only worked out twice. Tell the truth. Be supportive and encouraging — especially when new fitness goals are attained.

• Partners should have compatible schedules so that you can work out at the same times during the week. It's easier to stick to a set routine rather than to sporadic activities. Schedule your exercise sessions at the same time, on the same days. This is an excellent carrot to dangle in front of you and everyone on your team. Eventually, your workouts will become cemented into your daily routine.

• Everyone should be willing to work out at the same intensity levels — and not be afraid to sweat! Commit to gradually and progressively increasing your intensity.

Once you've put your team together, meet and map out your eight-week training schedule. Use your Athlete's Calendar to do this. Everyone should agree on this plan. Along with this, set your goals and share those goals with your partners.

Responsibilities Of Each Team Lean Partner

From the start, make sure everyone understands his or her responsibilities as a Team Lean partner. These will make your workouts safer and more productive.

• Be familiar with the proper use of all equipment and how to adjust it correctly.

• Wear proper workout clothes, including T-shirts or tank tops, leotards, sweat pants, and good-fitting shoes.

• "Spot" each other on certain weight training exercises. Spotting means monitoring a partner's exercise form, assisting with heavy lifts, catching missed lifts, communicating in advance with the lifter on how many reps will attempted, and keeping alert throughout the entire exercise sequence.

• Use safety equipment at all times, including collars and squat racks (a device that catches the barbell should a lifter not be able to finish a repetition).

• Know the limits of each partner.

• Return free weights to their proper location to prevent tripping hazards and keep the workout area clear of obstructions.

• Help each partner stay focused on the workout.

Choosing An Exercise Facility

If you or your partners are not already members of a gym, health club, or training facility, decide where you will train. Here are some key factors to consider:

• Cost. Membership fees should be affordable. Some facilities let you pay by the month — a good option since you can try the place out for a monthly fee before making a full commitment.

• Cleanliness. You can tell a lot about how a gym is managed by its housekeeping. Plates and weights should be put away and not scattered all over the floor. Equipment should be dust-free and well-maintained (no loose nuts and bolts, worn pulleys, torn padding, or broken weights).

• Variety of equipment. Check out the types of equipment available for exercises. A good facility will have a variety of barbells, dumbbells, machines, cable machines, and aerobic training equipment. A facility with an indoor running track gives you the option of doing your aerobics when there's inclement weather outside.

• Space. It's safer and more satisfying to work out in a spacious training environment, so you don't have to worry about bumping into machines and other exercisers, especially when you're training with your team. An ideal training facility is one where there's plenty of room between machines.

• Staff qualifications. A knowledgeable staff that is interested in your progress is a motivating factor. Find out what qualifications the staff has to manage the facility: degrees in exercise physiology or nutrition? certification through the American College of Sports Medicine or some other accrediting body? athletic accomplishments?

• Amenities. Showers, saunas, juice bars, massage therapy, and other health club amenities won't make you stronger or leaner, but they do convey a pleasant, client-oriented atmosphere. An important service to look for is fitness testing. That way, you can get your body fat measured easily and conveniently. If amenities are important to you, by all means look for a health club that offers them.

If you're uncomfortable with two or more of these factors, look elsewhere.

Keeping In Touch

You can also consider the Lean Bodies staff in Dallas as part of your extended Team Lean. If you have questions about working out or eating properly on the Lean Bodies program, call us at our special toll-free number. You'll be able to talk personally to one of our consultants.

At Lean Bodies, we're vitally interested in your health. So let us know how you're doing. Keep in touch with us. We're here to help you become the best you can be.

LEAN BODIES HOTLINE: 1-800-697-LEAN

23

More Motivation Tips

TO ACHIEVE the best shape of your life, you have to make a lifestyle change. The Lean Bodies Total Fitness program will help you achieve the next level of fitness. That's why before leaving the subject of exercise motivation, I want to give you some extra boosters to help you stay on track and reap all the benefits exercise offers.

Desire Personal Change

One of the most important initial exercise motivators is the desire for personal change. Perhaps you're unhappy with some present aspect of your health and conditioning. That's enough to get you going or to re-start a fitness effort that has somehow stalled. In one study, researchers watched 23 women who could attend a free aerobics class any time they wanted. The women most likely to attend the classes were the ones who were overweight, shorter, had several physical complaints, and felt anxious. The women knew exercise would provide some fairly rapid relief, so they took advantage of the classes and kept up their attendance.[1]

The lesson here: Nutrition and exercise strategies will solve your fitness problems. All you have to do is commit!

Select An Exercise Plan That's Fun

Exercising, then sticking to it, is much easier if you choose activities you can live with and love. When you start an exercise program, you typically view it as something to be tolerated — because it's "good for you." A better approach is to consider whether the exercise will achieve your fitness goals and be fun, to boot. Will you get to meet new people, learn some new skills, engage in some friendly competition? When shopping around for exercise, look at the quality of the exercise experience. Would you do it for a lifetime? You really have to love it that much.

Aerobics instructor and Lean Bodies participant Michelle D. offers this advice: "When you exercise, choose a type that you enjoy. If you don't enjoy it, you won't stick to it. Exercise you like well enough to continue is truly addicting."

If jogging isn't particularly your cup of tea, then find some other form of aerobics you like better. It's no use spending time at something you dislike. Not only that, it could be counterproductive, since you are apt to drop out. Experiment with different aerobic options.

As for weight training, it seems to be easier to stick to than other forms of exercises. In one study, adherence to a weight training program by women in their sixties was 83 percent. The reasons noted by researchers were that the women enjoyed weight training, and they lost body fat and got stronger while doing it.[2]

If you haven't started pumping iron yet, get moving — and learn as much about it as you can. With literally hundreds of exercises and routines you can do, and in hundreds of combinations, there's no way you can ever get bored with it.

Make Your Program Convenient

We're living in the "convenience age" — convenience stores, fast foods, one-stop shopping, and so forth. Exercise is no different. You're more likely to exercise if it's convenient to do so. In fact, studies have shown that one of the major reasons people drop out of exercise programs is inconvenience.

Join a gym that's close to your home or place of employment, so you can easily duck in for a workout. If your employer offers an on-site workout facility, sign up to use it. Another idea: Always carry a packed gym bag in your car so you'll be ready for your workout if you're out and about town.

Make Your Workouts Safe

Taking a tumble from a bicycle, twisting your ankle on a curb, dropping a dumbbell on your toe — these are just a few mishaps that can occur when you're not tuned into safety precautions for certain types of exercises. If you are not careful, accidents like these are enough to make you stop exercising for good! Make sure you are familiar with all the safety rules for each type of exercise you do.

Don't Overdo

Sometimes your enthusiasm for exercise can get the best of you, and you overdo a workout by exercising too hard, too long, or too many times in one week. Your muscles can get so stiff and sore that you wonder why you even bothered. Worse yet, there's the risk of injury. Any trauma to your bones, muscles, or connective tissue can potentially sideline you for a long time.

On the Lean Bodies Workout, the key is a gradual increase in intensity, duration, and frequency. Don't jump in at higher intensities right away. You're only asking for trouble if you do. Follow my guidelines for increasing intensity set forth in this book.

Get Family Support

There's a lot of data proving that people stay motivated to exercise when it's a family affair. Says Lean Body Sue S.: "Having someone do it with you really is one of the keys to keep going, plus being willing to change your lifestyle."

If your spouse or companion exercises regularly, then you are more likely to as well — and vice versa. Try to engender an attitude of fitness in your household, and everyone will get on the bandwagon.

Make A Financial Commitment

Gym owners can tell you plenty of stories about members who plopped down money for six- or 12-month contracts, but never again appeared after the first month. So it's hard to say whether making a financial commitment is really a good motivator. But, for some people it may be. In one study, exercisers committed to participating in a six-month aerobics program by paying $40 — which was reimbursable if they stuck with the program each week. Anyone who failed to work out weekly would lose the deposit. There was a control group who exercised but wasn't required to place the $40 deposit. Interestingly, the group which made the deposit had the best adherence — 97 percent, compared to the control group, whose adherence was only 19 percent. Exercisers who stuck to the program also had the best improvements in fitness levels, too.[3]

Hire A Personal Trainer

Many people who lack motivation or need one-on-one exercise instruction can find success in working with a personal trainer. Personal training fees can start from $20 an hour and go up from there, depending on where you live. Trainers will come to your home or work out with you at a gym or health club. They should help you with proper exercise form, assist you in reaching your goals, and motivate you to continue your exercise program.

Some questions to ask before you enlist the services of a personal trainer:

• Is the trainer certified? Certifications include those from the following groups: American College of Sports Medicine, National Strength and Conditioning Association, American Council on Exercise, and National Academy of Sports Medicine. Many personal trainers have degrees in physical education or exercise science — also a plus.

• Is the trainer knowledgeable in exercise, nutrition, and sports medicine?

• Does the trainer come highly recommended by other clients? Be sure to ask for references from past clients and employers.

• Does the trainer have an outgoing personality — in other words, is he or she someone you'd enjoy being around for a few hours a week? If a trainer lacks personality, chances are you won't want to stick with your program.

• Does the trainer have a fit physique? You certainly wouldn't hire a trainer who is pudgy with no muscle tone!

Here's a twist: Maybe some day you'll become a personal trainer! We've had Lean Bodies participants who got in such great shape that they wanted to share their success and knowledge with others by becoming personal trainers. Annette R. is a good example. She started the Lean Bodies program over a year ago and began to see results in just four months. Annette now competes in amateur bodybuilding contests and became certified as a personal trainer.

"I use only the Lean Bodies program with my clients," she says. "I also stress to each person that this program is not a diet, but a way of living a healthier life."

Annette has turned into a real motivator for her clients. She was kind enough to send us letters of thanks from her clients. Here's what they have to say:

• "I have lost 12 pounds, and the most important part of all this is that I feel so much better about myself. I have more energy, and my skin has improved 100 percent."

• "The nutritional weight loss program was terrific. Not only did I lose weight, I lost inches. I feel very good about myself and my appearance. In fact, my husband complimented me, which is unusual."

• "When I first started working with you to lose weight, I had my doubts, but nine months later and 75 pounds lighter, I feel like a whole new person. For the first time in my life, I can look in the mirror and actually feel good about what I see. I'm wearing clothes that I never thought I would be able to, and it's all because of the Lean Bodies program. I've taken the things that you've taught me and showed some other people how to eat. At first — like me — they thought I was nuts, but now they listen. My entire attitude toward food has changed. As for fast food, that now would be grilled chicken warmed up in the microwave, not a drive-through window."

Keep Your Program Goal-Oriented

Too often, decisions to start or re-start exercise are reactive, based on snap responses to negative situations. Your clothes are too tight, your spouse comments on the few extra pounds you've gained, or your doctor orders exercise for a medical condition. In reacting, you plunge into exercise, without a plan or strategy.

To succeed at exercise and to sustain motivation, you need an exercise plan designed around specific goals. As discussed in Chapter 6, draw up your goals and use your goal-setting form and Athlete's Calendar to help you achieve them.

Break The Age Barrier

Studies show that as people get older, they start to think that physical activity is both risky and inappropriate. Older adults typically underestimate their physical capabilities and fear exercise. In reality, there are few obstacles to exercise for healthy older adults and even more benefits. The research on how exercise, particularly weight training, is improving the quality of life for seniors could fill truckloads. If you think you're getting too old to exercise, let me tell you about my dad. He's 75 years old, squatting 200 pounds, and working on more!

Keep Your Program Effective

Gradual, incremental increases in intensity, frequency, and duration are the keys to losing fat, building lean mass, and staying in tip-top shape. The fact that you should make these upward adjustments — which mean working out harder — should not deter you from hanging in there. Look at them as challenges to be met, and you'll find yourself in a constant state of improvement. That's a motivator in itself!

Worth mentioning is that controversy does simmer over whether frequency and duration of exercise dampen willpower. One study indicates that it doesn't. Researchers put 33 non-exercising men and women into an exercise program to see what effects frequency and duration had on adherence. The result? No real effect.[4]

Reward Yourself

Whenever you achieve a goal, give yourself a reward — a new outfit, a special evening at your favorite restaurant, a weekend getaway. In other words, celebrate!

Rewards not only improve your motivation, they also enhance your fitness levels. Researchers at the University of Kentucky assigned 35 moderately fit people to one of three exercise groups: a self-monitoring group that kept written records; a reinforcement group that reported exercise progress verbally to another person who periodically handed out rewards; and a control group of sedentary subjects. The reinforcement/reward group had the most improvement in VO_2 max — an increase of 11 percent by the end of the 18-week study period, compared to a 5.3 percent increase among the self-monitoring exercisers.[5]

Vary Your Exercise Routine

Once you feel a routine has become stale, it is time to change. Experiment with other forms of exercise, new classes, different terrain on which to walk or jog.

Take A Cue From Athletes

If you want to stay in the best shape of your life (who doesn't?), then take a lesson from athletes. They prepare for a competition, an event, or a show by eating right and training regularly. By game time or show time, they're ready.

Do you have a "show" or a "game" coming up, like a high school reunion or a summer vacation? Adopt the athlete's mentality and start "training" for it. What you're really doing is setting short-term goals to achieve long-term fitness.

Don't Stop

Any lapse in your exercise routine can really throw you out of whack, physically and mentally. It's that much harder to get back in the swing of things after a layoff. You feel as though you've taken some giant steps backward. Here's a look at what happens:

• Muscles decrease in size, tone, and strength.

• There's a shift toward more fast-twitch fibers (that's the kind that doesn't burn fat well.)

• The activity of fat-burning enzymes declines.

• Your muscles lose their ability to store energy-yielding glycogen. Stop working out for a month, and your muscle glycogen could drop by 40 percent![6]

• The heart becomes de-conditioned quite rapidly, and VO_2 max declines.

• You lose speed and flexibility.

• Body fat piles back on, and fat cells enlarge.

Make the Lean Bodies Workout your lifestyle, and the health benefits keep rolling in. A case in point: Researchers in Denmark studied 118 older women who were overweight to see what effect long-term exercise had on health and body composition. Six months earlier, the women had completed a 12-week program in which they were assigned to a diet-only group, an exercise group, or a control group. The women from the exercise group who continued to work out after the study had lost more overall body-weight than the non-exercisers (nearly 24 pounds compared to 14.5 pounds). Also, the exercisers pared their fat pounds significantly, losing an average of 22 pounds of pure fat, compared to 12 pounds for the non-exercisers. One other benefit of staying on the move: The exercisers' resting metabolic rate was the highest among all the groups.[7]

This study is a good reminder for all of us: To keep the fat off, we've got to keep moving.

And once you make Lean Bodies your lifestyle, you are likely to make other health-promoting lifestyle changes, too. We've seen people stop smoking, change their diets for good, reduce the stress in their lives, and more.

24

Epilogue: Your New Lifestyle

YOU ARISE in the morning, feeling ready to bound from bed after a sound night's sleep. This morning, like so many mornings, a brisk walk is on the agenda for keeping your metabolism revved up all day. Slipping into your walking gear, you catch a look at your physique in the mirror. Lean, muscularly fit. You haven't looked that good in years. It's a look and a feel you want to keep.

Out the door, you greet the day energetically. Before long, your brisk walk turns into a nice jog. Your heart is pounding at a good pace, and you can almost feel your body tapping into fat for fuel. Periodically, you check your heart rate to make sure you're working within your target range. You are, and that's a good sign. As great as the morning jog is, the anticipation of a big breakfast awaits at the end of the line.

By breakfast, your body tanks are ready to be filled with clean-burning fuel — pure, close-to-nature carbs, lean proteins, and other nutrient-packed food. Hot, steaming oatmeal with some other whole grains stirred in. A tall glass of vitamin-rich vegetable juice. Scrambled egg whites with chunks of non-fat smoked turkey mixed in for extra flavor. All washed down with cold, refreshing spring water.

Next, you are off to work. Your physical and mental productivity still amazes you. You run circles around everyone in the office. No more mid-morning or mid-afternoon slumps. It's like you're turbocharged. The more you get done, the faster the day goes. The only clockwatching you do is to see when it's time to eat your next meal.

But then there are the stares and the offhand comments when you break out your huge amounts of food at mid-morning, lunch, and mid-afternoon. Like the one from your boss yesterday: "You're going to get big as a house, eating that much."

You smile, roll up your sleeve, and flex your biceps. "I hope so" is your reply. Or perhaps you flip out your before-and-after pictures as proof of what can be accomplished by eating more, not less.

But for every disparaging remark, there are two or three uplifting comments. "You look great." "You've really trimmed down." "You glow all over."

Of course, many people want to know what the "hitch" is — how can you eat so much and look so fit? You tell them, and this fuels their fire to get started on a lifestyle change.

After work, some of your co-workers are headed home to the couch, but you are on your way to the gym. The anticipation of your workout pumps you up mentally before you even hit the door.

There's one thing about the gym you love even more than the workout itself — the camaraderie of the people who care about their personal fitness as much as you do. Surrounding yourself with fitness-minded people provides constant support and encouragement.

Today, you're working out with two of those people — the members of your Team Lean. Throughout the next 45 minutes, you'll coach each other to achieve heavier poundages, higher intensities, and ultimately, even better levels of fitness.

You love lifting the weights and seeing your well-defined muscles ripple with each movement. This isn't narcissism; it's gratitude, especially when you remember your formally fat, sluggish self. You're glad those days are behind you.

After each set, you record your poundages in your notebook. This is an important practice, since it lets you exceed previous records from workout to workout.

For you and your two partners, there are more compliments from people in the gym. Your team has become a motivating force for others around it.

You decide to finish off your weight training workout with some heart-pumping aerobics. You have more than enough energy to push to the max.

At home that evening, you're ready for another Lean Bodies meal — grilled chicken breast, a cinnamon-baked sweet potato, a salad that's overflowing with fresh veggies. Early on the program, you changed your mind-set toward food. Now you think of it primarily as fuel. Nonetheless, it still tastes incredible all the time.

With another great day almost finished, you are ready for tomorrow. No longer do you have to wish for a healthy, fit body. You've got it, and you intend to keep it.

This is your healthy and fit lifestyle, now that you are living the Lean Bodies way, or is it? I want to challenge you right now to put into action the principles covered in this book. Read and re-read the testimonials and case studies it contains. Their reports provide evidence for everyone, including you, that the Lean Bodies programs can produce dramatic results, starting right now and continuing for a lifetime when you stick with them.

You now have everything you need to know to develop the fit,

firm, healthy body you've always wanted — and keep it that way.
You can do it!

Appendices

What About Me? Help For Hard Gainers

What About Me? Help For Hard Gainers

NOT EVERYONE WANTS TO LOSE body fat. Many people are more interested in gaining weight. Maybe you're one of them. You're already lean — too lean, in fact. Your body resembles a straight pin. No matter what you do, you can't put on weight — you are what we call a "hard gainer." Does this mean you are forever destined to be thin and lanky?

Not at all. Believe me, I can empathize with you. I'm a formerly too-thin guy also. I used to weigh a skinny 120 pounds, with virtually no muscle mass to speak of.

But today at age 41, I have gained 25 pounds of lean muscle.

But enough about me. What about you? Can you transform your body, too? You bet. In working with hard gainers, I recommend that they follow four basic principles: consume more calories, spread throughout the day; choose growth-producing foods; use supplements to increase calories; and adhere to a program of weight training designed to build lean mass.

1. Consume more calories, spread out through the day.

Have you ever cared for a new puppy? If you have, you know that it has to be fed six or more times a day. When you do, it's ravenous for the chow. That's because the puppy is in a growth mode.

So are you, if your goal is to put on weight. You must eat more food, and it must be divided into six or more feedings a day, spaced two or three hours apart. Begin to gradually increase your calories every few days (not weekly as we recommended for people trying to lose body fat). It takes 2,500 calories to build a pound of muscle so you should try to gradually build up to that extra amount.

Contrary to what you might think, you won't put on body fat by eating more food. A gradual increase of calories from the right foods keeps that from happening.

2. Eat growth-producing foods.

A problem many hard gainers have is that their metabolisms run high all the time. You burn up food as fast as you consume it. Research has found that fast-metabolizers do well on a diet that's high in carbohydrates — unlike slower metabolizers, who do better on fewer carbs.

Using the Lean Bodies program, you may want to adjust your carbohydrate intake upward — to 65 to 70 percent of your daily calories. Your carbohydrates should come from starchy carbs and fibrous vegetables — at a ratio of two to one (two servings of starchy carbs for every one serving of fibrous carbs). Starchy carbohydrates include whole grains, beans, legumes, potatoes, yams, brown rice, and any natural, unrefined carbohydrate source. Fibrous vegetables include salad vegetables, broccoli, cauliflower, green beans, carrots, green leafy vegetables, among others.

Increasing your carb intake is not done at the expense of protein, however. Protein should comprise 20 to 25 percent of your daily calories. Also, very convincing research exists showing that muscle-gaining individuals should eat 1 to 1.25 grams of protein per pound of bodyweight each day to support tissue growth. Your proteins should of the low-fat variety. The best protein choices are white meat poultry, fish, egg whites, and lean red meat. Certain starchy vegetables like beans, legumes, and corn contain protein, too, and this should be taken into consideration when figuring your daily protein allowance for your bodyweight.

Be sure to combine your foods properly, too. Always eat protein with carbohydrates to allow for a steady, even release of energy.

Include in your daily diet some essential fatty acids (EFAs) as well. EFAs are made up of compounds called linoleic acid, linolenic acid, and arachidonic acid, all contained primarily in vegetable oils. Omega-3 fatty acids are another type of EFA, and they are found in fish. All EFAs are vitamin-like substances that have a protective effect on the body. Hard gainers should take in up to 1 tablespoon of EFAs a day. Good sources are safflower oil, canola oil, flaxseed oil, and sunflower seed oil.

For more information on proper diet planning, refer to the first Lean Bodies book.

3. Supplement for extra calories.

One way to increase your calories is through the use of supplements — MCT oil and protein/carbohydrate supplements, in particular. MCT oil contains 114 calories per tablespoon and thus is an excellent way to add in extra calories. Two ounces of a protein/carbohydrate supplement mixed with water after each meal adds approximately 1,260 calories, depending on which product you use. As you can see, it's not that difficult to boost your daily calories.

4. Follow a weight training program geared for growth.

Hard gainers benefit most from weight training routines in which basic exercises, heavy weights, and low-to-moderate repetitions are employed. In other words, don't hit the gym every day and do a lot of exercises and reps.

Here's an example of a routine that should produce significant muscular gains:

*Three-Day-A-Week Routine For Hard Gainers
Monday/Wednesday/Friday

Muscle Groups	Exercise	Sets/Repetitions
Legs	Squat or Leg Press	3 - 4 sets of 8 - 12 reps
Chest	Barbell Bench Press	3 - 4 sets of 8 - 12 reps
Back	Front Pulldown	3 - 4 sets of 8 - 12 reps
Shoulders	Barbell Shoulder Press	3 - 4 sets of 8 - 12 reps
Biceps	Barbell Curl	3 - 4 sets of 8 - 12 reps
Triceps	Close-Grip Bench Press	3 - 4 sets of 8 - 12 reps
Calves	Standing Calf Raise	2 sets of 10 - 12 reps
Abdominals	Body Crunch With Weight	12 - 15 reps

* Be sure to warm up with 10 minutes of mild aerobics or by performing a very light warmup set before each exercise.

After you feel like you've gained some muscle mass on the above routine, switch to one of the split routines described in this book. Using a split routine will help you better isolate and develop muscle groups.

As for aerobics, you need this form of exercise to build and maintain aerobic fitness, as well as to create extra capillaries for better delivery of nutrients to muscle cells for growth. My recommendation for hard gainers is to do aerobics three times a week, gradually increasing intensity, for 20 to 30 minutes each time. Make sure you're eating enough to fuel your body for exercise and daily activities.

Making Progress

Keep track of your gains, too. If you're not gaining muscle, you may have to concentrate on increasing your calories even more for a few weeks. Try working out at higher intensities, too, with heavier weights. You may want to experiment with advanced techniques such as negatives and supersets to force your body back into a growth mode. These techniques are covered in Chapter 12.

If I can transform my skinny physique, so can you. Just stay dedicated and consistent, and the label "hard gainer" will be a thing of the past.

Ask Cliff: Questions And Answers About The Lean Bodies Workout

Ask Cliff: *Questions And Answers About The Lean Bodies Workout*

Why doesn't dieting work?

Nearly 95 percent of those who go on low-calorie diets regain their weight, plus interest, within five years. Low-calorie diets slow the metabolism. One reason is that up to 50 percent of the weight you lose on a diet is muscle. Since "muscle is metabolism," losing it slows your metabolism.

Also, once you start eating normally again, your body accelerates its buildup of fat as if to prepare for the next "famine" (another diet). This famine/fat acceleration cycle makes you regain more body fat after each period of dieting.

Other factors are at work to keep you fat. Did you know, for example, that by not eating, you are training your body to store fat? Here's why: Cut calories and your body is tricked into thinking it's starving. A special fat storage enzyme goes to work, signalling your body to stockpile fat once it's fed again.

Did you also realize that diets are hazardous to your health? We now know that dieters have higher rates of heart disease, diabetes, and osteoporosis, the loss of vital bone mineral. Dieting can also cause loss of brain tissue. Plus, on-again/off-again dieting accelerates the degeneration of the body.

Now that I've become more active on the Lean Bodies Workout, should I eat more protein?

More and more, research in clinical nutrition is showing that active people, including athletes, have increased requirements for protein — far above the current RDA of 0.8 grams/kg bodyweight per day for the average person. Unfortunately, the RDA was developed from studies of sedentary individuals and doesn't take into account the needs of more active people. If you are active, 20 to 25 percent of your daily caloric intake should come from lean protein. This amount should provide ample "building material" for the repair and recovery processes that take place following exercise. You can't grow muscles if you don't feed them properly.

I've always heard that active people need to concentrate on filling up with carbohydrates, yet you seem to emphasize protein. What gives?

Too much carb in the diet can hinder fat loss, particularly if you're not very active. A carb overload can trigger a high release of the hormone insulin into the bloodstream. Insulin activates fat cell enzymes, facilitating the movement of fat from the bloodstream into fat cells for storage. Additionally, insulin prevents glucagon (a hormone that opposes the action of insulin) from entering the bloodstream, and glucagon is responsible for unlocking fat stores. The cumulative result of these interactions is the ready conversion of carbs to body fat. If you reduce your carb consumption, you inhibit the release of insulin. This in turn stimulates glucagon, the hormone that helps liberate fat stores. Manipulation of carbs in this manner is one way to promote fat loss.

I'm not a proponent of low-carb, high-protein diets, however. If you cut your carbs too much, you risk running low on energy. Most active people find that they do best on a diet in which at least 60 to 65 percent of the total calories come from complex carbs such as those recommended on the Lean Bodies eating program.

With all the talk about carbs, protein has gotten lost in the shuffle, when in fact it may be the most important nutrient for controlling weight and developing lean mass. People who already have fast metabolisms do better with a higher carb diet, but slow metabolizers — those who need to lose body fat — do better by concentrating on protein. The key is to balance insulin and glucagon, and you can do this by consuming a diet consisting of 20 to 25 percent protein, 60 to 65 percent carbs, and the rest from fat.

Do I need to take supplements on the Lean Bodies program?

Not necessarily. Food comes first. Once you're eating properly, you may want to take supplements just as extra insurance that you're getting all the nutrients you need. Supplements are an excellent way to increase the nutrients you need for growth, repair, and good health. Also, supplements are a convenient way to prepare mock meals.

Should I eat during a workout?

If you're fueling yourself well throughout the day, I see no need to consume anything — except water (four to six ounces every 15 minutes). Many people on the Lean Bodies Workout have achieved extra energizing results by sipping a ProCarb™ drink during their workouts. This is an easily digested carbohydrate supplement. See the Appendix C for more information.

Is weight training done just to look good, or does it have some health benefit?

Weight training does as much on the inside as it does on the outside — perhaps more. As you'll discover in the lesson on exercise, weight training keeps your body youthful, no matter what your age; boosts your fat-burning potential; keeps your heart, bones, and muscles healthy; and much more.

A former weight training skeptic turned Lean Body, Teri D. has this to say about weight training: "It has given me a body I would never have dreamed of in terms of being lean and hard. My muscles are well-defined. I weigh as much as I ever have, but I wear the smallest size I ever have. The results have been dramatic."

How exactly does weight training burn fat?

Weight training turns up your metabolism by developing calorie-burning, metabolically active muscle. Muscle is your metabolism. The muscle you gain directly boosts your metabolic rate so you can burn more fat, even in your sleep.

I'm a vegetarian. Can I still build muscle on the Lean Bodies Workout?

Yes, but you have to concentrate on getting adequate amounts of protein. Vegetarians who eat eggs and milk (lacto-ovo vegetarians) are getting quality protein in their diets; they just have to eat more of those foods to do so. If you've cut out all animal proteins, you have more of a challenge on your hands. In that case, you have to eat a lot of high-protein vegetable foods, such as beans, legumes, soy products, and whole grains. These foods contain only limited proportions of the eight essential amino acids, the protein sub-units that must be supplied from food. Your body can't make them on its own.

This is not a problem if you properly combine your vegetarian foods, however, to balance out the essential amino acids. What one food lacks in terms of a certain amino acid, another food supplies. The combination of beans and rice, for example, is a good way to get the right balance of amino acids in a meal.

Won't weight training bulk me up?

No. The word "bulk" refers to fat over muscle. With weight training, you're building muscle, not fat. It's extremely difficult to build big muscles, contrary to what you might think. But you can do it more rapidly and effectively with a nutrient-dense eating program, intense weight training, and aerobic exercise. Together, these components will result in a gain of lean mass and a reduction in body fat.

How many times a week should I weight train to see results?

On the Lean Bodies Workout, you weight train your entire body only twice a week. This is enough to see measurable results within several weeks. Also, this is the amount of weight training recommended by the American College of Sports Medicine (ACSM).

You can also use a "split routine" — dividing your body up into sections and working them on different days. Regardless of what routine you use — full body or split system — make sure you exercise each muscle group twice a week. That's all it takes to firm up and gain strength.

If I lift weights fast, will I burn more fat?

Not at all. In fact, you'll risk injuring your joints and other connective tissue. An injury like that could put you out of commission for a while. You won't burn any fat sitting at home!

The best technique for moving weights is in a slow, controlled action on both the lifting and lowering phase of an exercise. This builds calorie-burning, body-firming muscle best. The firmer your body, the faster it burns fat.

Do I need to do my weight training exercises in a certain order?

Definitely. Always exercise your larger muscle groups first, since they place greater energy demands on your body. In certain large-muscle exercises, smaller muscles are called into play to assist. For that reason, you don't want to tire those smaller muscles too early in your workout or you won't have enough strength to really push hard on your larger-muscle exercises.

Which are better for getting results — free weights or exercise machines?

Anything — even your own bodyweight — will work, as long as you work out intensely. It's not the machine, the barbell, or the dumbbell that's producing the muscle-shaping, muscle-toning results. It's the effort you put behind the equipment!

About halfway through my weight training workout, I seem to poop out. Why is that?

Right off the bat, I'd say nutrition. You need to re-analyze your diet: Are you eating at least five meals a day? Are you fueling yourself properly with the right kinds of proteins and carbohydrates? Have you increased your calories to match the increases in your exercise intensity? Have you tried nutritional supplementation for extra calories and health protection?

During your workouts, you may want to try sipping a serving of ProCarb™ (see Appendix C for information). Doing so can give you a constant supply of liquid food fuel and keep your energy levels high. Also, make sure you're getting adequate rest and sleep.

If you honestly feel as though you're doing everything right nutritionally and getting enough rest during the week, then you may need to consult your physician to explore possible non-nutritional reasons for your tiredness.

Will I lose flexibility if I weight train?

Flexibility is the ability to move a muscle easily through its full range of motion. Many of the most flexible athletes in the world use weight training in their workouts. Performed properly, weight training should improve your flexibility. You might try some stretching exercises following your weight training workout to enhance your flexibility as well.

As a woman, I'm afraid to pursue weight training. Won't I build bulky muscles?

No! The reason men build bulk is because their bodies are naturally loaded with testosterone, a hormone that develops sex characteristics, including large muscles. Women have minute quantities of this hormone, but not enough for huge muscle-building.

Women also have smaller muscle fibers than men do — another reason you won't build muscular bulk. What you will build, however, is beautifully shaped, well-toned muscles. One more thing: Weight training favorably stresses bone, and bone density increases as a result. This offers a protective effect against bone-crippling osteoporosis in later years.

Why is it so hard for women to get rid of the fat on their legs and hips?

The activity of the fat-promoting enzyme lipoprotein lipase is very high in the thighs and hips of women, so a lot of fat is stored there. Women actually need these stores to prepare for pregnancy and lactation. Regardless, you can still whittle down your thighs and hips. It takes consistent weight training, high-intensity aerobics, and a nutrient-dense, protein-rich diet, as recommended by the Lean Bodies eating program. I can't emphasize protein enough. Let me relate a story that most women find very motivating.

One of my clients had always race-walked for 45 minutes each day while following a low-calorie diet. Even so, her muscles still lacked tone. She wasn't taking in enough protein to rebuild muscle in the recovery period following exercise. Her muscles were in a perpetual state of breakdown. After three weeks on the program, she flexed her legs for us. Her quadriceps and calves were lean and hard, all because she was getting enough protein to build lean tissue.

But back to weight training for a moment: Make sure you are working your legs and hips three times a week for best results. Also, consider progressing to some of the advanced workout techniques suggested in Chapter 12 to take care of these trouble spots.

Will muscle turn to fat if I stop working out?

No. A muscle fiber, which is actually a cell, can't magically transform into a fat cell. They're physiologically different. However, if you stop training, your muscle cells will shrink, and your fat cells will expand.

What are the other health benefits derived from weight training other than increased strength and improved metabolism?

Widely accepted research has shown that weight-bearing exercise builds bone density, cardiac health, lung health, to name just a few. See Chapter 3 for a rundown of weight training's many other health benefits.

Which type of aerobic exercise is best for burning fat?

Any type in which you gradually increase your intensity and enjoy pursuing.

I'm really afraid to try running. Haven't people died while running?

Deaths due to heart attacks have occurred during exercise, but they are rare. Even so, they make headlines. One study of cardiovascular complications among YMCA exercisers found one death per 2,897,057 person-hours and one non-fatal cardiac arrest per 2,253,267 person-hours.[1] Running and other forms of aerobics are associated more with the prevention of heart disease.

According the medical experts, deaths during aerobic exercise occur when there is disease present, although it often goes undetected. Some causes include: irregular heartbeat as a result of clogged arteries, enlarged diseased heart (usually an inherited condition), a family history of heart disease, an aneurysm in the aorta, or any underlying heart disease in which symptoms have gone ignored. Anyone who exercises should have a physical examination first. Seek medical advice immediately if you experience any possible heart-related symptoms.

How long will it take me to start getting stronger?

As quickly as your second weight training workout!

I had a heart attack several years ago. Should I even exercise?

First things first: Consult your cardiologist. If exercise is prescribed, make sure that you are closely monitored by a medical team.

Physicians do put heart patients in cardiac rehabilitation programs that involve exercise, both weight training and aerobics. By building strength and muscular endurance, weight training helps a patient return to daily work and recreational activities after a cardiac incident. Both weight training and aerobics have been shown to produce favorable outcomes on heart health in terms of controlling cholesterol, decreasing blood pressure, reducing body fat, and managing stress. There's some evidence that exercise may reduce the chance of a second heart attack.

Won't exercise make me hungry?

Possibly — but what's wrong with that? Remember, on the Lean Bodies eating program, you should be gradually increasing your calories.

In reality, exercise (especially intense exercise) acts like an appetite suppressant, usually for the first few hours after working out. There are several possible reasons for this. First, exercise increases catecholamines (epinephrine and norepinephrine), and these are appetite suppressants. Second, exercise elevates body temperature — a condition that squelches desire for food. Likewise, working out in hot weather can suppress the appetite.

Is it okay to run in hot weather?

If your body isn't accustomed to exercising in the heat, there are some risks to doing so, including heat cramps, heat exhaustion, and heat stroke. Heat cramps can occur in exercising muscles as a result of electrolyte and water losses through sweat.

Excessive losses reduce blood volume. Your cardiovascular system then works overtime to dispatch blood to the skin, muscles, and other needy places. Your body can't cool off because the distribution of blood is poor. Heat exhaustion can then set in. Symptoms include tiredness, dizziness, fainting, vomiting, low blood pressure, and a weak pulse.

Push yourself beyond that point, and you can suffer heat stroke, a life-threatening condition requiring immediate medical treatment. With heat stroke, your body's heat-regulating mechanisms fail, and the result is a dangerously high fever, usually exceeding 104° F. Besides the high fever, other symptoms of heat stroke include hot and dry skin, rapid pulse and breathing, high blood pressure, confusion and unconsciousness.

You can train your body to exercise in hot environments without risk, however. Work out in the heat for up to an hour each day for about a week, but do so at lower intensities. It takes only a week to 10 days for your body to fully adapt to working out in the heat. Also, fill up on starchy carbs during this time in order to pack away more muscle glycogen. This is important, since exercising in the heat uses up more glycogen. Later, when your body gets used to the heat, it won't use as much glycogen. Be sure to supplement with minerals and electrolytes, too, to prevent losses of these important nutrients.

A man exercising in the heat can lose up to two quarts of sweat in an hour. Not rehydrating yourself can spell danger. On days when you're training in the heat, drink 10 or more cups of water throughout the day, including while you're working out.

The company where I work offers a worksite wellness program. I'm thinking about signing up. Is this a good idea, or should I do something on my own?

I believe in the value of such programs. As part of a study, Lean Bodies is conducting such a program for a corporation in Texas, and the results among participants as of this writing have been phenomenal.

The worksite is considered the ideal place for getting people to start a regular exercise program. However, studies show that half of the people who start such programs drop out within a year or less. Be sure to thoroughly check out the program your company offers. Is the exercise facility well-equipped and professionally staffed? Can you conveniently participate in it? Does it provide good instruction and education on nutrition and exercise? Are there incentives for meeting exercise and fitness goals? What health assessment services are available? Can spouses and family members participate, too? These are just a few points to consider before signing up.

Your company can provide the best wellness program around, but unless the participants commit to getting in shape, it's all for naught. Becoming more active and changing your diet requires dedication and discipline. You've got to be willing to go the distance. The worksite wellness program provides the vehicle for change, but you're the one who makes the changes happen.

I'm starting the Lean Bodies Workout after not exercising for about a year. What advice can you give me?

Getting back into action after a layoff is known as "retraining." A year is a rather long time, and you may have lost quite a bit of conditioning. I recommend that you start at a low-intensity level and progress gradually — as if you were just starting out — in both aerobics and weight training. Be sure to warm up and cool down during each exercise session. Above all, don't try to tackle your pre-layoff poundages or aerobic intensities. You'll only set yourself up for injury — and possibly another layoff. Also, be sure to get enough rest to allow your muscles and entire body to recuperate fully. Follow the Lean Bodies eating program to help you regain your energy levels and to push your body's growth and repair mechanisms.

I've never done aerobic exercise before. How soon can I expect changes in my resting heart rate?

Research with sedentary individuals shows that they have an average resting heart rate of 80 to 100 beats per minute. Assuming you fit in that category, your heart rate should drop by one beat each week the first few weeks of starting an aerobic exercise program. After eight weeks of aerobic training, expect your heart rate to decrease from 80 to 72 beats a minute.[2] Keep records of heart rate during rest and exercise to make sure positive changes are occurring in your cardiovascular health.

Appendix C

Recommended Products

Recommended Products

Skinfold calipers for measuring body fat and lean mass: An accurate tool for measuring body fat using skinfold calipers is the Parrillo Performance BodyStat Kit.

Vitamins: Parrillo Performance Essential Vitamin Formula™

Minerals: Parrillo Performance Mineral-Electrolyte Formula™

Carotenoids: NeoLife Carotenoid Complex

Branched-chain amino acids: Parrillo Performance Muscle Amino Formula™

Lipotropics: Parrillo Performance Advanced Lipotropic Formula™

Carbohydrate supplements: Parrillo Performance ProCarb™

Protein supplements: Parrillo Performance Hi-Protein Powder™, Vita-Herb Protein Powder, and Beverly International 100% Egg White Protein Powder

Sports nutrition bar: Parrillo Performance Supplement Bar

Omega-3 fatty acids: NeoLife Salmon Oil

MCT Oil: Parrillo Performance CapTri®

Evening primrose oil: Efamol

CoQ$_{10}$: Twin Labs Coenzyme 10

Chromium: Twin Labs Chromium Picolinate

Desiccated liver: Parrillo Performance Liver Amino Formula™

Please note: Parrillo Performance supplements may be ordered by calling Lean Bodies at **1-800-697-LEAN.** Other supplements can be found at most health food stores or sports nutrition centers.

Appendix D

Recommended Reading

Recommended Reading

Cliff Sheats' Lean Bodies: The Revolutionary Approach To Losing Body Fat By Increasing Calories by Cliff Sheats and Maggie Greenwood-Robinson (The Summit Publishing Group, Warner Books).

Cliff Sheats' Lean Bodies Cookbook by Cliff Sheats and Linda Thornburgh (The Summit Publishing Group, Warner Books).

High Performance Bodybuilding by John Parrillo and Maggie Greenwood-Robinson (Perigee Books).

John Parrillo's 50 Workout Secrets by John Parrillo and Maggie Greenwood-Robinson (Perigee Books).

Pain-Free: The Definitive Guide to Healing Arthritis, Low-Back Pain, and Sports Injuries Through Nutrition and Supplements by Luke Bucci, Ph.D. (The Summit Publishing Group).

Dr. Bob Arnot's Guide To Turning Back The Clock by Robert Arnot, M.D. (Little & Brown).

A Glossary Of Terms Used In The Lean Bodies Workout

A Glossary Of Terms Used In

The Lean Bodies Workout

Actin and myosin. Two contractile proteins in muscle that slide over each other like two pieces of a telescope to cause contraction.

ATP (adenosine triphosphate). A molecular fuel that makes muscles contract, conducts nerve impulses, and promotes other cellular energy processes.

Aerobics. Continuous action exercise that can be performed within the body's ability to use and process oxygen. Examples include walking, jogging, running, cycling, swimming, and cross-country skiing.

Amino acids. The basic building blocks of protein used for growth and maintenance of body tissues.

Anaerobic exercise. Effort characterized by brief bursts of work, such as weight training or sprinting. Anaerobic exercise creates an oxygen debt in which the body can't keep up with the oxygen demands of exercising muscles.

Anemia. Low levels of hemoglobin in the blood.

Antioxidants. Vitamins, minerals, and enzymes that fight free radicals and protect the body from disease.

Atherosclerosis. A condition in which the arteries become clogged and narrowed by a buildup of cholesterol and other materials in the inner arterial walls.

Barbell. A long bar with adjustable weights or plates at each end.

Basal metabolic rate. The minimum energy required to maintain life processes while the body is at rest.

Biotin. A B-complex vitamin involved in the metabolism of fats.

Body composition. A health-related factor in fitness that describes the relative percentages of body fat, muscle, bone, and water in the body.

Body fat. Stored fat which is usually deposited around the hips, thighs, and abdomen.

Branched-chain amino acids. A trio of amino acids — leucine, valine, and isoleucine — whose chief role is to assist the muscles in synthesizing other amino acids for growth and repair.

Cables. Weight training equipment with pulleys attached to adjustable weight stacks.

Calipers. A special instrument that measures the amount of fat just under the skin.

Calorie. Unit of energy available from food.

Calorie cost. The number of calories burned to produce energy for a specific activity or exercise.

Carbohydrates. Foods that serve as the main energy source for the body. Examples include whole grains, legumes, vegetables, and fruits.

Cardiovascular fitness. The ability of the heart and blood vessels to adequately circulate blood and oxygen throughout the body.

Carnitine. A protein-like nutrient that shuttles fat in the form of fatty acids — essential fuel for the body — into the mitochondria of cells to be burned for energy.

Catecholamines. The hormones epinephrine and norepinephrine. Secreted by the brain, catecholamines drive metabolic processes.

Cell. The smallest structure in the body.

Cholesterol. A fatty substance found in some foods and manufactured by the body for many vital functions.

Choline. Present in all living cells, choline is considered a member of the vitamin B-complex family. As a lipotropic, it works to prevent fat from building up in the liver and facilitates the transfer of fat into cells to be burned for energy.

Chondroitin sulfates. Compounds found naturally in cartilage and other connective tissues.

Chondroprotective agents. A class of nutrients that stimulates the repair of cartilage, a plastic-like tissue found throughout the body.

Chromium. A trace nutrient essential for normal sugar and fat metabolism.

Coenzyme Q$_{10}$. A compound directly involved in energy-producing reactions that ultimately generate ATP, the molecular fuel for cells. It resides in the mitochondria and membranes of cells.

Contraction. Bending or flexing of the muscle.

Cool-down. A gradual reduction of exercise intensity towards the end of a workout. A cool-down lets physiological processes return to normal.

Cortisol. A hormone released during exercise that frees up amino acids to be used in the liver to produce glucose.

Creatine. A constituent of muscles that assists in the transfer of energy in muscle cells and in the production of ATP for muscular contractions. Creatine is available as a nutritional supplement.

Creatine phosphate (CP). A compound that can supply energy for a few short seconds of work.

Desiccated liver. A concentrated form of beef liver that has been processed to remove the cholesterol but to preserve the nutrient content of the liver.

Dumbbell. A short bar with adjustable or fixed plates on each end.

Duration. The length of time that exercise is performed.

Electrolytes. Minerals that are responsible for maintaining the fluid balance inside and outside cells.

Enzyme. A protein which brings about chemical changes without being affected itself.

Epinephrine. A hormone that triggers the breakdown of muscle glycogen into glucose and stored fat into fatty acids.

Essential fatty acids (EFAs). Vitamin-like substances that have a protective effect on the body. They are called essential because the body cannot manufacture them. They must be obtained from food.

Exercise. Structured, repetitive bodily activity designed to improve muscle tone, cardiovascular fitness, and other components of physical conditioning.

Exercising heart rate. The rate at which your heart beats during exercise.

Failure. The point in an exercise at which you can no longer do any more work.

Fast-twitch fiber. A type of muscle fiber that contracts quickly and is called into play during intense, short-burst activities like weight training. Also called Type II fiber.

Fatigue. A loss of power to continue exercising or performing an activity.

Fats. Foods that provide energy for the body. Examples include vegetable oil and margarine.

Fiber. Indigestible portion of plant foods that has many health benefits.

Fibrils. Structures that form muscle fibers.

Flexibility. The range of motion of a joint.

Forced reps. An advanced weight training technique in which your partner helps you perform additional repetitions after you've reached failure.

Form. Exercise style.

Free fatty acids (FFA). Blood-borne fat.

Free radicals. Unstable molecules that destroy cells and cause disease.

Free weights. Barbells and dumbbells.

Frequency. The number of times you exercise weekly.

Fructose. A sugar found in fruit and fruit juices.

General warmup. Mild, whole-body exercise that elevates muscle temperature to get ready for a workout.

Generic equipment. Exercise benches, slant boards, and chinning bars.

Giant set. A grouping of four or five exercises for the same muscle, performed in sequence without rest in between.

Glucagon. As glucose levels dip, this hormone is secreted to raise them. This hormone is also responsible for unlocking fat stores under certain dietary conditions.

Glucosamine. A type of sugar molecule manufactured naturally by cartilage cells from glucose and the amino acid, glutamine.

Glucose. Blood sugar.

Glycogen. Carbohydrate stored in the liver and muscles.

Glycolosis. The breakdown of glycogen into glucose so that cells can make ATP.

Glycolytic energy system. The sequence of events that converts glycogen into energy for the body.

Growth hormone. A chemical that stimulates growth from birth to adolescence and has other functions later in life, including roles in fat-burning and muscle-building.

Heart rate. The number of times a heart beats per minute.

HDL (high density lipoprotein). A type of cholesterol in the blood that has a protective effect against the buildup of plaque in the arteries.

Heme iron. Iron found in animal protein.

Hemoglobin. A protein in red blood cells that transports oxygen from the lungs to the rest of the body.

Hormones. Chemicals in the body that control various physiological processes.

Hyperplagia. The addition of more muscle fibers, and a theory of muscle growth.

Hypertrophy. Increase in the size of muscle fibers.

Hypoglycemia. Low blood sugar.

Immune system. A complex network of various types of cells and organs that work together to fight disease, from the common cold to deadly cancers.

Inositol. A B-complex vitamin and lipotropic that helps prevent dangerous accumulations of fat in the arteries and keeps the liver, heart, and kidneys healthy.

Insulin. A hormone that decreases blood glucose levels by moving glucose into cells to be used for fuel and increases the rate at which glucose is converted to glycogen. Insulin also promotes amino acid uptake by muscle cells and encourages the storage of excess calories as body fat.

Intensity. The degree of effort exerted in exercise.

Interval. The rest period between each repeat (lap or time sequence) in interval training.

Interval training. Alternately speeding up and slowing down during aerobic exercise.

Joint. The intersection of two bones.

Lean mass. The amount of muscle on your body.

Ligaments. Fibrous bands of tissue that connect bones at joints.

Lipoprotein lipase (LPL). An enzyme governing fat storage. Repetitive low-calorie dieting causes the body to produce more LPL, and more body fat is produced and stored as a result.

Lipotropic. A fat-burning agent.

Low density lipoproteins (LDL). A type of cholesterol in the blood. High levels contribute to coronary heart disease.

Lymphocytes. A type of white blood cell formed in the lymphatic system. About 20 to 30 percent of the white blood cells in the body are lymphocytes.

Maximum heart rate (MHR). The highest heart rate at which a person's heart can beat. MHR is calculated by subtracting your age from 220.

Medical history. A list of your past illnesses, present health conditions, symptoms, risk factors, and medications you're taking. This history is used by your physician to determine the state of your health and to see if you're at risk for any diseases.

MCT oil (medium chain triglyceride oil). A dietary fat metabolized in such a way that very little is stored as body fat.

Metabolic rate. The speed at which your body burns calories.

Metabolism. The physiological process that converts food to energy so that your body can function.

Mineral. Inorganic nutrients needed by the body for a wide range of enzymatic and metabolic functions.

Mitochondria. The energy factory of cells where nutrients are burned for energy.

Muscle. Body tissue composed of threadlike fibers that contract and relax.

Muscular endurance. The ability of a muscle to repeat contractions without fatiguing.

Muscle fibers. Threadlike structures in the muscles that are actually cells.

Muscular strength. The amount of external force a muscle can exert.

Negatives. The lowering portions of a weight training exercise.

Non-heme iron. Type of iron found in plants.

Norepinephrine. A hormone that triggers the breakdown of muscle glycogen into glucose and fat into fatty acids for use by muscle cells.

Omega-3 fatty acids. Essential fats found in fish that appear to prevent blood clots and the buildup of plaque on arterial walls. Omega-3 fatty acids also play a role in strengthening the immune system.

Osteoporosis. An age-related reduction in bone mineral that leads to crippling fractures, and sometimes death. Usually affects postmenopausal women.

Oxygen energy system. Sequence of events in which oxygen is processed with nutrients to create energy for the body.

Phosphagen energy system. One of the energy systems of the body. It supplies creatine phosphate for short bursts of muscular activity.

Plates. Disc-shaped weights used on barbells, dumbbells, and plate-loading machines.

Plate-loading machine. A type of equipment in which poundage changes are made by loading plates onto a bar on the machine. The leg press is a good example of a plate-loading machine.

Progressive overload. Continually putting more demands on your muscles than they're used to.

Protein. Food group necessary for growth and repair of body tissues.

Radial pulse. The pulse taken at the wrist.

Range of motion. The full path of an exercise, from extension to contraction and back again.

Recommended Dietary Allowances (RDA). A technical standard established by the National Research Council of the National Academy of Sciences that sets forth the amount of vitamins and minerals needed by the body to maintain good health.

Repeat. A concept used in interval training that describes a specific distance like a lap or a specific time.

Repetition. In weight training, the number of times an exercise is performed. In interval training, the number of times you perform each repeat.

Resistance. The weight of a barbell, dumbbell, or one's own bodyweight.

Routine. A grouping of exercises.

Set. A series of repetitions.

Slow-twitch fiber. A type of muscle fiber that contracts slowly and is used in endurance-type exercises. Also known at Type I fiber.

Split routine. In weight training, a system of dividing the body into muscle groups and exercising those groups on different days.

Spotter. A training partner who helps in the performance of an exercise.

Superset. An advanced weight training technique that combines two or more exercises, performed right after each other with no rest in between.

Supplementation. The use of vitamins, minerals, and other nutrients as nutritional adjuncts to the diet.

Target heart rate (THR). The heart rate at which you try to exercise.

Temporal artery. A site at the front of the ear at which the pulse can be taken to determine heart rate.

Tendons. Fibrous bands of tissue that connect muscle to bones.

Testosterone. A hormone responsible for the development of male sex characteristics.

Thermogenesis. The production of body heat — a process that increases oxygen consumption and boosts the metabolic rate.

Triglycerides. The storage form of fat.

Trisets. Three exercises for the same muscle group performed in succession without rest in between.

Very low density lipoprotein. A harmful type of cholesterol.

Vitamins. Organic substances found in food that perform many vital functions in the body.

VO₂ max. The body's oxygen-processing capacity, usually expressed in percentages.

Weight stack machine. Weight training equipment that employs a stack of weights that can be adjusted to give you the poundage you want to lift. Adjustments are made by inserting a pin into the stack. Leg curl and leg extension machines are examples of weight stack machines.

Weight training. The use of barbells, dumbbells, machines, and other forms of resistance to develop muscle and strength.

References

References

Chapter 1: The Five Exercise Secrets for Fat Loss

1. J. P. McCarthy, J. C. Agre, B. K. Graf, M. A. Pozniak, and A. C. Vailas, "Compatibility of Adaptive Responses With Combining Strength and Endurance Training," *Medicine and Science in Sports and Exercise* 27, no. 3 (March 1995): 429-436.

Chapter 2: Lean Bodies Aerobics — The Benefits

1. M. Bricklin, "Good News: Dieting Is Dead," *Prevention* (October 1993): 39-40, 113.

2. University of Victoria, "Cycling Fat," *Canadian Journal of Sports Science* 13, no. 4: 204-207.

3. S. Shinkai, S. Watanbe, Kurokawa, and J. Torii, et al, "Effects of 12 Weeks of Aerobic Exercise Plus Dietary Restriction On Body Composition, Resting Energy Expenditure and Aerobic Fitness In Mildly Obese Middle-Aged Women," *European Journal of Applied Physiology* 68, no. 3 (1994): 258-265.

4. P. A. Mole, "Impact of Energy Intake and Exercise on Resting Metabolic Rate," *Sports Medicine* 10, no. 2 (August 1990): 72-87.

5. J. H. Wilmore and D. L. Costill, *Physiology of Sport and Exercise* (Champaign, Illinois: Human Kinetics, 1994), 436.

6. W. D. McArdle, F. I. Katch, and V. L. Katch, "Body Composition, Energy Balance, and Weight Control," in *Exercise*

Physiology: Energy, Nutrition, and Human Performance, 3rd ed. (Philadelphia: Lea & Febiger), 628.

7. Wilmore and Costill, *Physiology of Sport and Exercise,* 481.

8. H. L. Nash, "Re-emphasizing the Role of Exercise in Preventing Heart Disease," *The Physician and Sportsmedicine* 17, no. 3 (March 1989): 219-225.

9. R. Stamler, J. Stamler, F. C. Gosch, et al., "Primary Prevention of Hypertension by Nutritional Hygienic Means. Final Report of a Randomized, Controlled Trial," *Journal of the American Medical Association* 262 (1989): 1801-1807. Reported by K. Thompson in *The Physician and Sportsmedicine* 18, no. 2 (February 1990): 19-20.

10. B. Bassett, "Ten Great Excuses for Starting An Exercise Program," *Bestways* (October 1984): 1.

11. A. LaPerriere, M. H. Antoni, G. Ironson, A. Perry, et al., "Effects of Aerobic Exercise Training on Lymphocyte Subpopulations," *International Journal of Sports Medicine* 15, Supplement 3 (October 1994): 8127-8130.

12. Nehlsen-Cannarella, D. C. Neiman, A. J. Balk-Lamberton, P. A. Markoff, et al., "The Effects of Moderate Exercise Training On Immune Response," *Medicine and Science in Sports and Exercise* 23, no. 1 (January 1991): 64-70.

13. E. R. Eichner, "Infection, Immunity, and Exercise: What To Tell Patients," *The Physician and Sportsmedicine* 21, no. 1 (January 1993): 125-135.

14. International Society of Sport Psychology, "Physical Activity and Psychological Benefits," *The Physician and Sportsmedicine* 20,

no. 10 (October 1992): 179-184.

15. J. Dua and L. Hargreaves, "Effect of Aerobic Exercise On Negative Affect, Positive Affect, Stress, and Depression," *Perceptual Motor Skills* 75, no. 2 (October 1992): 355-361.

Chapter 3: Lean Bodies Weight Training — The Benefits

1. M. S. Treuth, A. S. Ryan, R. E. Pratley, M. A. Rubin, et al., "Effects of Strength Training On Total and Regional Body Composition in Older Men," *Journal of Applied Physiology* 77, no. 2 (August 1994): 614-620.

2. S. Siplia and H. Suominen, "Effects of Strength and Endurance Training On Thigh and Leg Mass Muscle and Composition in Elderly Women," *Journal of Applied Physiology* 78, no. 1 (January 1995): 334-340.

3. C. Melby, C. Scholl, G. Edwards, and R. Bullough, "Effect of Acute Resistance Exercise On Postexercise Energy Expenditure of Metabolic Rate," *Journal of Applied Physiology* 75, no. 4 (October 1993): 1847-1853.

4. A. Benaidy, N. Davis, E. Delgado, S. Garcia, and E. Al-Herzalia, "Effects of a Job-Simulated Exercise Programme On Employees Performing Manual Handling Operations," *Ergonomics* 37, no. 1 (January 1994): 95-106.

5. H. S. Milner-Brown, "Muscle Strengthening In a Post-Polio Subject Through a High-resistance Weight-training Program," *Archives of Physical Medicine and Rehabilitation* 74, no. 11 (November 1993): 1165-1167.

6. F. Taylor, "Building Bones With Bodybuilding," *The Physician and*

Sportsmedicine 19, no. 3 (March 1991): 51.

7. M. K. Karlsson, O. Jonnell, and K. J. Obrant, "Bone Mineral Density in Weight Lifters," *Calcification Tissue International* 52, no. 3 (March 1993): 212-215.

8. R. C. Handy, J. S. Anderson, K. E. Whalen, and L. M. Harvill, "Regional Differences in Bone Density of Young Men Involved in Different Exercises," *Medicine and Science in Sports and Exercise* 26, no. 7 (July 1994): 884-888.

9. L. Goldberg, D. L. Elliot, R. W. Schutz, and F. E. Kloster, "Changes In Lipid and Lipoprotein Levels After Weight Training," *Journal of the American Medical Association* 252, no. 4 (July 27, 1984): 505-506.

10. B. F. Hurley, J. M. Hagberg, A. P. Goldberg, D. R. Seals, et al., "Resistive Training Can Reduce Coronary Risk Factors Without Altering VO₂ Max or Percent Body Fat," *Medicine and Science in Sports and Exercise* 20, no. 2 (April 1988): 150-154.

11. T. L. Dupler and C. Cortes, "Effects of a Whole-body Resistive Training Regimen in the Elderly," *Gerontology* 39, no. 6 (1993): 314-319.

Chapter 4: The Intensity Factor In Fat-Burning

1. Wilmore and Costill, *Physiology of Sport and Exercise,* 228 (see Ch. 2, n. 5).

2. Ibid., 177.

4. L. L. Hinkleman and D. C. Nieman, "The Effects of a Walking Program On Body Composition and Serum Lipids and Lipoproteins in Overweight Women," *Journal of Sports Medicine and Physical Fitness* 33, no. 1 (March 1993): 49-58.

5. A. E. Hardman, P. R. Jones, N. G. Norgan, and A. Hudson, "Brisk Walking Improves Endurance Fitness Without Changing Body Fatness in Previously Sedentary Women," *European Journal of Applied Physiology* 65, no. 4 (1992): 354-359.

6. C. Pollack, "Does Exercise Intensity Matter?" *The Physician and Sportsmedicine* 20, no. 12 (December 1992): 123-126.

7. L. Schnirring, "Exercise Benefits Build With Intensity," *The Physician and Sportsmedicine* 23, no. 2 (February 1995): 21.

8. A. Tremblay, J. P. Despres, C. Leblanc, C. L. Craig, et al., "Effect of Intensity of Physical Activity On Body Fatness and Fat Distribution," *American Journal of Clinical Nutrition* 51, no. 2 (February 1990): 153-157.

Chapter 5: How Your Body Responds To The Lean Bodies Workout

1. *The Illustrated Encyclopedia of the Human Body* (New York: Exeter Books, 1984): 39.

2. Wilmore and Costill, *Physiology of Sport and Exercise,* 147.

3. L. B. Oscai and W. K. Palmer, "Discussion: Adipose Tissue Adaptation to Exercise," in *Exercise, Fitness, and Health* (Champaign, Illinois: Human Kinetics Books, 1988): 325-328.

4. W. J. Gonyea, D. G. Sale, F. B. Gonyea, and A. Mikesky, "Exercise Induced Increases in Muscle Fiber Number," *European Journal of Applied Physiology* 55, no. 2 (1986): 137-141.

Chapter 6: Getting Started

1. B. A. Franklin, R. F. DeBusk, N. F. Gorson, P. Hanson, and M.

L. Pollock, "Exercise Testing Update," *The Physician and Sportsmedicine* 12, no. 12 (December 1991): 111-120.

Chapter 9: Lean Bodies Exercise Routines
2. M. J. Gibala, J. D. MacDougall, M. A. Tarnopolsky, W. T. Stauber, and A. Elorriaga, "Changes In Human Skeletal Muscle Ultrastructure and Force Production After Acute Resistance Exercise," *Journal of Applied Physiology* 78, no. 2 (February 1995): 702-708.

Chapter 10: Your Best Aerobic Bets
1. Roundtable discussion, "Walking for Fitness," *The Physician and Sportsmedicine* 14, no. 10 (October 1986): 145-159.

2. Ibid.

3. Ibid.

4. D. C. Nieman, *Fitness and Sports Medicine: An Introduction* (Palo Alto, California: Bull Publishing Co., 1990): 424.

5. W. D. McArdle, F. I. Katch, and V. L. Katch, *Exercise Physiology: Energy Nutrition, and Human Performance*, 2nd ed. (Philadelphia: Lea & Febiger, 1986): 157.

Chapter 11: 10 Ways To Become A Better Fat-Burner
1. O. Anderson, "Burn, Baby, Burn," *Runner's World* (May 1995): 38.

2. E. M. Gorostiaga, C. B. Walter, C. Foster, and R. C. Hickson, "Uniqueness of Interval and Continuous Training at the Same Maintained Exercise Intensity," *European Journal of Applied Physiology* 63, no. 2 (1991): 101-107.

3. D. T. Martin, J. C. Scifres, S. D. Zimmerman, and J. G. Wilkinson, "Effects of Interval Training and a Taper On Cycling Performance and Isokinetic Leg Strength," *International Journal of Sports Medicine* 15, no. 8 (November 1994): 485-491.

Chapter 15: Say Goodbye To Fatigue

1. Wilmore and Costill, *Physiology of Sport and Exercise*, 114 (see Ch. 2, n. 5).

2. Ibid.

3. Ibid., 150-151.

4. J. E. Donnelly, J. Jakicic, and S. Gunderson, "Diet and Body Composition. Effect of Very Low Calorie Diets and Exercise," *Sports Medicine* 12, no. 4 (October 1991): 237-249.

5. A. Burfoot, "The Brain Connection," *Runner's World* (August 1994): 70-75.

Chapter 17: Nutrient Protectors

1. P. M. Clarkson, "Antioxidants and Physical Performance," *Critical Review of Food Science Nutrition* 35, nos. 1-2 (1995): 131-141.

2. M. Meydani, W. J. Evans, G. Handelman, L. Biddle, et al., "Protective Effect of Vitamin E On Exercise-induced Oxidative Stress," *American Journal of Physiology* 264, no. 5 part 2 (May 1993): R992-998.

3. A. Hartmann, A. M. Niess, M. Grunert-Fuchs, and G. Speit, "Vitamin E Prevents Exercise-induced DNA Damage," *Mutation Research* 346, no. 4 (April 1995): 195-202.

4. P. Shimer, "Vitamin C Protects Muscles," *Runner's World* (August 1994): 22.

5. L. Bucci, *Nutrients As Ergogenic Aids for Sports and Exercise* (Boca Raton: CRC Press, 1993): 67-68.

6. M. Murakoshi, J. Takayasu, O. Kimura, E. Kohmura, et al., "Inhibitory Effects of Alpha Carotene On Proliferation of the Human Neuroblastoma Cell Line," *Journal of the National Cancer Institute* 81, no. 21 (November 1, 1989): 1649-1652.
Also: M. Murakoshi, H. Nishino, Y. Satomi, J. Takayasu, et al., "Potent Preventive Action of Alpha Carotene Against Carcinogenesis: Spontaneous Liver Carcinogenesis and Promothing State of Lung and Skin Carcinogenesis In Mice Are Suppressed More Effectively by Alpha-Carotene Than By Beta Carotene," *Cancer Research* 52, no. 23 (December 1, 1992): 6583-6587.

7. R. Ziegler, L. Brinton, P. Nasca, et al., "Diet and the Risk of Vulvar Cancer," *American Journal of Epidemiology* 132 (1990): 778.

8. "Dietary Carotenoids, Vitamins A, C, E, and Advanced Age Related Macular Degeneration," *Journal of the American Medical Association* 272, no. 18 (1994): 1413-1420.

9. G. Comstock, K. Helzlsouuer, and T. Bush, "Prediagnostic Serum Levels of Carotenoids and Vitamin E As Related to Subsequent Cancer in Washington, Maryland," *American Journal of Clinical Nutrition* 53 (1991): 260s-264s.

10. E. Dixon, B. J. Burri, A. Clifford, et al., "Effects of a Carotene-deficient Diet On Measures of Oxidative Susceptibility and Superoxide Dismutase Activity in Adult Women," *Free Radical Biology & Medicine* 17 (1994): 537-544.

11. T. R. Kramer, B. J. Burri, and T. R. Neidlinger, "Carotenoid-Flavenoid Modulated Immune Response in Women," *FASEB Journal* 9, no. 3 (1995): A170.

12. L. R. Brilla and T. F. Haley, "Effect of Magnesium Supplementation On Strength Training in Humans," *Journal of the American College of Nutrition* 11, no. 3 (June 1992): 326-329.

13. R. L. Prince, M. Smith, I. M. Dick, R. I. Price, et al., "Prevention of Postmenopausal Osteoporosis. A Comparative Study of Exercise, Calcium Supplementation, and Hormone-replacement Therapy," *New England Journal of Medicine* 24325, no. 17 (October 24, 1991): 1189-1195.

14. L. C. Pacelli, "To Fortify Bones Use Calcium and Exercise," *The Physician and Sportsmedicine* 7, no. 11 (November 1989): 27-28.

15. L. Bucci, *Pain-Free: The Definitive Guide to Healing Arthritis, Low-Back Pain, and Sports Injuries Through Nutrition and Supplements* (The Summit Publishing Group, 1995): 74.

Chapter 18: Energy Optimizers

1. A. K. Lindeman, "Eating for Endurance or Ultraendurance," *The Physician and Sportsmedicine* 20, no. 3 (March 1992): 87-101.

2. E. F. Coyle and E. Coyle, "Carbohydrates That Speed Recovery From Training," *The Physician and Sportsmedicine* 21, no. 2 (February 1993): 111-123.

3. C. M. Maresh, L. E. Armstrong, J. R. Hoffman, D. R. Hannon, et al., "Dietary Supplementation and Improved Anaerobic Performance," *International Journal of Sport Nutrition* 4 (1994): 387-397.

4. P. D. Balsom, K. Soderlund, and B. Ekblom, "Creatine in Humans With Special Reference to Creatine Supplementation," *Physiology III* 18, no. 4 (October 1994): 268-280.

5. D. A. MacLean, T. E. Graham, and B. Saltrin, "Branched-chain Amino Acids Augment Ammonia Metabolism While Attenuating Protein Breakdown During Exercise," *American Journal of Physiology* 267, no. 6 part 1 (December 1994): E1010-1022.

6. E. Blomstrand and E. A. Newsholme, "Effect of Branched-chain Amino Acid Supplementation On the Exercise-induced Change in Aromatic Amino Acid Concentration in Human Muscle," *Acta Physiologica Scandinavica* 146, no. 3 (November 1992): 293-298.

7. G. Carli, M. Bonifazi, L. Lodi, C. Lupo, et al., "Changes in Exercise-induced Hormone Response to Branched Chain Amino Acid Administration," *European Journal of Applied Physiology* 64, no. 3 (1992): 272-277.

8. H. Yamabe and H. Fukuzaki, "The Beneficial Effect of Coenzyme Q_{10} On the Impaired Aerobic Function in Middle Aged Women Without Organic Disease," in *Biomedical and Clinical Aspects of Coenzyme Q_{10}*, vol. 6, eds. K. Folers, T. Yamagani, and G. P. Littarru (Amsterdam: Elsevier, 1991): 521. Reported in L. Bucci, *Nutrients As Ergogenic Aids for Sports and Exercise* (Boca Raton: CRC Press, 1993): 55.

9. P. Zeppilli, B. Merlino, A. DeLuca, et al., "Influence of Coenzyme Q_{10} On Physical Work Capacity in Athletes, Sedentary People and Patients With Mitochondrial Disease," in Biomedical and Clinical Aspects of *Coenzyme Q_{10}*, vol. 6, eds. K. Folers, T. Yamagani, and G. P. Littarru (Amsterdam: Elsevier, 1991): 521.

Reported in L. Bucci, *Nutrients As Ergogenic Aids for Sports and Exercise* (Boca Raton: CRC Press, 1993): 55.

10. E. Madio, R. Palermo, G. Reloni, and G. P. Littarru, "Effect of CoQ₁₀ Administration in High Level Athletes," in Biomedical and Clinical Aspects of *Coenzyme* Q₁₀, vol. 6, eds. K. Folers, T. Yamagani, and G. P. Littarru (Amsterdam: Elsevier, 1991): 521. Reported in L. Bucci, *Nutrients As Ergogenic Aids for Sports and Exercise* (Boca Raton: CRC Press, 1993): 56.

Chapter 19: Lipotropics For Mobilizing Fat

2. G. I. Dragan, A. Vasiliu, E. Georgescu, and N. Eremia, "Studies Concerning Chronic and Acute Effects of L-Carnitina in Elite Athletes," *Physiologie* 26, no. 2 (April-June 1989): 111-129.

3. G. I. Dragan, W. Wagner, and E. Ploesteanu, "Studies Concerning the Ergogenic Value of Protein Supply and L-Carnitine in Elite Junior Cyclists," *Physiologie* 25, no. 3 (July-September 1988): 129-132.

4. C. De Simone, M. Ferrari, A. Lozzi, D. Meli, et al., "Vitamins and Immunity: Influence of L-Carnitine on the Immune System," *Acta Vitamino Enzymol* 4, nos. 1-2 (1982): 135-140.

5. L. Vaughn, "Discovering the Healing Powers of Carnitine," *Prevention* (October 1994): 50-54.

6. P. M. Clarkson, "Nutritional Ergogenic Aids: Carnitine," *International Journal of Sports Medicine* 2 (1992): 185-190.

7. R. A. Anderson, "Essentiality of Chromium in Humans," *Scientific Total Environment* 86, nos. 1-2 (October 1989): 75-81.

8. W. W. Campbell and R. A. Anderson, "Effects of Aerobic

Exercise and Training On the Trace Minerals Chromium, Zinc, and Copper," *Sports Medicine* 4, no. 1 (January-February 1987): 9-18.

9. A. S. Kozlovsky, P. B. Moser, S. Reiser, and R. A. Anderson, "Effects of Diets High in Simple Sugars On Urinary Chromium Losses," *Metabolism* 35, no. 6 (June 1986): 515-518.

10. E. Mazer, "Biotin – The Little Known Lifesaver," *Prevention* (July 1981): 97-102.

Chapter 20: Special Lipids For Exercisers

1. J. E. Kinsella, "Dietary Fish Oils," *Nutrition Today* (November-December 1986): 7-14.

2. B. Sears, *BIOSYN Training Manual* (Marblehead, Massachusetts: BIOSYN), in L. Bucci, *Nutrients As Ergogenic Aids For Sports and Exercise* (Boca Raton: CRC Press, 1993): 19-20.

3. L. R. Brilla and T. E. Landerholm, "Effects of Fish Oil Supplementation and Exercise On Serum Lipids and Aerobic Fitness," *Journal of Sports Medicine* 30, no. 2 (1990): 173, in L. Bucci, *Nutrients As Ergogenic Aids For Sports and Exercise* (Boca Raton: CRC Press, 1993): 19-20.

4. L. Bucci, *Nutrients As Ergogenic Aids For Sports and Exercise* (Boca Raton: CRC Press, 1993): 19-20.

Chapter 21: Desiccated Liver

1. T. Swinney, "Liver: The Premium Energy Food," *Ironman* (November 1991): 52.

2. M. J. Aquado, M. S. Romero, J. A. Moreno, F. Fernandez, and M. Gutierrez, "Reduction of Iron Deposits After Physical Exercise of Short Duration," *Sangre* 37, no. 6 (December 1992): 425-427.

3. A. Cordova Martinez and J. F. Escanero, "Iron, Transferrin, and Haptoglobin Levels After a Single Bout of Exercise in Men," *Physiological Behavior* 51, no. 4 (April 1992): 719-722.

4. W. Schobersberger, M. Tschann, W. Hasibeder, M. Steidl, et al., "Consequences of Six Weeks of Strength Training on Red Blood Cells O_2 Transport and Iron Status," *European Journal of Applied Physiology* 60, no. 3 (1990): 163-168.

6. S. S. Harris, "Helping Active Women Avoid Anemia," *The Physician and Sportsmedicine* 23, no. 5 (May 1995): 35-46.

Chapter 22: Team Lean: A Revolutionary New Motivational Concept

1. J. I. Robison and M. A. Rogers, "Adherence to Exercise Programmes. Recommendations," *Sports Medicine* 17, no. 1 (January 1994): 39-52.

2. A. C. King, C. B. Taylor, W. L. Haskell, and R. F. Debusk, "Strategies for Increasing Early Adherence to and Long-term Maintenance of Home-based Exercise Training in Healthy Middle-aged Men and Women," *American Journal of Cardiology* 61, no. 8 (March 1, 1988): 628-632.

3. P. A. Gillett, "Self-reported Factors Influencing Exercise Adherence in Overweight Women," *Nurs Res* 37, no. 1 (January-February 1988): 25-29.

4. B. E. Stoffelmayr, B. E. Mavis, T. Stachnik, J. Robison, et al., "A

Program Model to Enhance Adherence in Work-site-based Fitness Programs," *Journal of Occupational Medicine* 34, no. 2 (February 1992): 156-161.

Chapter 23: More Motivation Tips

1. E. A. Klonoff, A. Annechild, and H. Landrine, "Predicting Exercise Adherence in Women: The Role of Psychological and Physiological Factors," *Preventive Medicine* 23, no. 2 (March 1994): 257-262.

2. J. F. Nichols, D. K. Omizo, K. K. Peterson, and K. P. Nelson, "Efficacy of Heavy-resistance Training for Active Women Over Sixty: Muscular Strength, Body Composition, and Program Adherence," *Journal of the American Geriatric Society* 41, no. 3 (March 1993): 205-210.

3. J. I. Robison, M. A. Rogers, J. J. Carlson, B. E. Mavis, et al., "Effects of a Six-month Incentive-based Exercise Program on Adherence and Work Capacity," *Medicine and Science in Sports and Exercise* 24, no. 1 (January 1992): 85-93.

4. S. A. White, R. V. Croce, E. M. Louriero, and N. Vroman, "Effects of Frequency and Duration of Exercise Sessions on Physical Activity Levels and Adherence," *Perceptual Motor Skills* 73, no. 1 (August 1991): 172-174.

5. M. P. Noland, "The Effects of Self-monitoring and Reinforcement on Exercise Adherence," *Research Quarterly for Exercise and Sports* 60, no. 3 (September 1989): 216-224.

6. Wilmore and Costill, *Physiology of Sport and Exercise*, 311 (see Ch. 2, n. 5).

7. O. L. Svendsen, C. Hassager, and C. Christiansen: "Six Months' Follow-up on Exercise Added to Short-term Diet on Overweight Postmenopausal Women – Effects on Body Composition, Resting Metabolic Rate, Cardiovascular Risk Factors and Bone," *International Journal of Obesity Related Metabolic Disorders* 18, no. 10 (October 1994): 692-698.

Appendix B: Ask Cliff: Questions And Answers About the Lean Bodies Workout

1. D. C. Nieman, *Fitness and Sports Medicine: An Introduction*, 435 (see Ch. 10, n. 4).

2. Wilmore and Costill, *Physiology of Sport and Exercise*, 220 (see Ch. 2, n. 5).

Authors' Biographies

Authors' Bi

CLIFF SHEATS is a clinical nutritionist and the creator and author of CLIFF SHEATS' LEAN BODIES and THE LEAN BODIES COOKBOOK.

He appears frequently as a guest expert on radio and television talk shows. In addition, he writes columns on nutrition for fitness publications, consults with amateur and professional athletes, and is involved in clinical research on nutrition.

Cliff has his bachelor of science degree in sports administration and nutrition, and his master of science degree in sports administration. He has worked in clinical practice with the medical profession (cardiology), specializing in nutrition. He is currently involved in a research doctorate program in London, England. Cliff is a Fellow in Good Standing with the American Council of Applied Clinical Nutrition, a member of the International and American Associations of Clinical Nutritionists (IAACN), and a member of the Royal Society of Health. Cliff is also a certified tennis professional with the United States Professional Tennis Registry USA.

ographies

MAGGIE GREENWOOD-ROBINSON is the co-author of five other fitness books: BUILT! The New Bodybuilding For Everyone, CLIFF SHEATS' LEAN BODIES, HIGH-PERFORMANCE BODYBUILDING, JOHN PARRILLO'S 50 WORKOUT SECRETS, and NUTRITION FOR AN ACTIVE LIFETIME.

Her articles have appeared in *Women's Sports and Fitness*, *Working Woman*, *Muscle and Fitness*, *Female Bodybuilding*, and many other publications. In addition, she has taught bodyshaping classes at the University of Southern Indiana and is preparing to volunteer as an exercise trainer in an inner-city ministry. Maggie is currently working on an exercise book for women.

Index

Index